Surgical Decision Making, Evidence, and Artificial Intelligence

Editors

JASON BINGHAM
CARLY ECKERT
MATTHEW ECKERT

SURGICAL CLINICS OF NORTH AMERICA

www.surgical.theclinics.com

Consulting Editor
RONALD F. MARTIN

April 2023 • Volume 103 • Number 2

ELSEVIER

1600 John F. Kennedy Boulevard • Suite 1800 • Philadelphia, Pennsylvania, 19103-2899

http://www.surgical.theclinics.com

SURGICAL CLINICS OF NORTH AMERICA Volume 103, Number 2
April 2023 ISSN 0039–6109, ISBN-13: 978-0-323-93979-9

Editor: John Vassallo
Developmental Editor: Hannah Lopez

Surgical Clinics of North America (ISSN 0039–6109) is published bimonthly by Elsevier Inc., 360 Park Avenue South, New York, NY 10010-1710. Months of publication are February, April, June, August, October, and December. Business and Editorial Offices: 1600 John F. Kennedy Blvd., Suite 1800, Philadelphia, PA 19103-2899. Periodicals postage paid at New York, NY and additional mailing offices. Subscription prices are $479.00 per year for US individuals, $1045.00 per year for US institutions, $100.00 per year for US & Canadian students and residents, $575.00 per year for Canadian individuals, $1327.00 per year for Canadian institutions, $580.00 for international individuals, $1327.00 per year for international institutions and $250.00 per year for foreign students/residents. To receive student/resident rate, orders must be accompanied by name of affiliated institution, date of term, and the *signature* of program/residency coordinator on institution letterhead. Orders will be billed at individual rate until proof of status is received. Foreign air speed delivery is included in all *Clinics* subscription prices. All prices are subject to change without notice. POSTMASTER: Send address changes to *Surgical Clinics*, Elsevier Health Sciences Division, Subscription Customer Service, 3251 Riverport Lane, Maryland Heights, MO 63043. **Customer Service (orders, claims, online, change of address): Telephone: 1-800-654-2452 (U.S. and Canada); 314-447-8871 (outside U.S. and Canada). Fax: 314-447-8029. E-mail: journalscustomerservice-usa@elsevier.com (for print support); journalsonlinesupport-usa@elsevier.com (for online support).**

Reprints. For copies of 100 or more, of articles in this publication, please contact the Commercial Reprints Department, Elsevier Inc., 360 Park Avenue South, New York, New York 10010-1710. Tel. 212-633-3874, Fax: 212-633-3820, E-mail: reprints@elsevier.com.

Surgical Clinics of North America is also published in Spanish by McGraw-Hill Interamericana Editores S.A., P.O. Box 5-237 06500 Mexico D.F. Mexico; and in Portuguese by Interlivros Edicoes Ltda., Rua Comandante Coelho 1085, CEP 21250, Rio de Janeiro, Brazil; and in Greek by Paschalidis Medical Publications, Athens Greece.

Surgical Clinics of North America is covered in *MEDLINE/PubMed (Index Medicus)*, *EMBASE/Excerpta Medica*, *Current Contents/Clinical Medicine*, *Current Contents/Life Sciences*, *Science Citation Index*, and *ISI/BIOMED*.

Contributors

CONSULTING EDITOR

RONALD F. MARTIN, MD, FACS
Colonel (Retired), United States Army Reserve, Department of General Surgery, Pullman Surgical Associates, Pullman Regional Hospital and Clinic Network, Pullman, Washington

EDITORS

JASON BINGHAM, MD, FACS
Associate Professor of Surgery, Chief, Uniformed Services University of Health Sciences, Bethesda, Maryland; Chief, General Surgery, Madigan Army Medical Center, Tacoma, Washington

CARLY ECKERT, MD, MPH
Department of Epidemiology, University of North Carolina, Chapel Hill, North Carolina; University of Washington School of Public Health, Department of Epidemiology, Seattle, Washington

MATTHEW ECKERT, MD, FACS
Associate Professor, Uniformed Services University of Health Sciences, Bethesda, Maryland; Assistant Professor, Acute Care Surgery, Department of Surgery, The University of North Carolina at Chapel Hill, Chapel Hill, North Carolina

AUTHORS

MUSTAFA ABID, MD
Department of Surgery, Resident Surgeon, The University of North Carolina at Chapel Hill, Chapel Hill, North Carolina

JASON BINGHAM, MD, FACS
Associate Professor of Surgery, Chief, Uniformed Services University of Health Sciences, Bethesda, Maryland; Chief, General Surgery, Madigan Army Medical Center, Tacoma, Washington

RACHEL CALLCUT, MD, MSPH, FACS
Division Chief, Trauma, Acute Care Surgery and Surgical Critical Care, University of California, Davis, Sacramento, California

SAMUEL P. CARMICHAEL II, MD, MS
Assistant Professor, Department of Surgery, Wake Forest School of Medicine, Winston-Salem, North Carolina

LEO ANTHONY CELI, MD, MPH, MSc
Principal Research Scientist, Laboratory of Computational Physiology, Massachusetts Institute of Technology, Cambridge, Massachusetts; Associate Professor of Medicine, Beth Israel Deaconess Medical Center, Boston, Massachusetts

JODI CRAMER, BA, JD, LLM
Attorney, United States Coast Guard, Washington, DC

LESLY A. DOSSETT, MD, MPH
Associate Professor, Department of Surgery, Michigan Medicine, Ann Arbor, Michigan

MOLLY J. DOUGLAS, MD, FACS
Clinical Assistant Professor, Department of Surgery, University of Arizona, Tucson, Arizona

CARLY ECKERT, MD, MPH
Department of Epidemiology, University of North Carolina, Chapel Hill, North Carolina; University of Washington School of Public Health, Department of Epidemiology, Seattle, Washington

HEATHER L. EVANS, MD, MS
Professor, Vice Chair of Clinical Research and Applied Informatics, Department of Surgery, Medical University of South Carolina, Charleston, South Carolina

STEFAN D. HOLUBAR, MD, MS, FACS
IBD Surgery Section Chief, Director of Research, Department of Colon and Rectal Surgery, Digestive Disease and Surgery Institute, Cleveland Clinic, Cleveland, Ohio

TASHA M. HUGHES, MD, MPH
Assistant Professor, Department of Surgery, Michigan Medicine, Ann Arbor, Michigan

DAVID M. KLINE, PhD
Assistant Professor of Biostatistics and Data Science, Division of Public Health Sciences, Department of Biostatistics and Data Science, Wake Forest School of Medicine, Winston-Salem, North Carolina

DANIEL LAMMERS, MD
Department of General Surgery, Madigan Army Medical Center, Tacoma, Washington

EDDY P. LINCANGO, MD
Research Fellow, Department of Colon and Rectal Surgery, Digestive Disease and Surgery Institute, Cleveland Clinic, Cleveland, Ohio

JOHN MCCLELLAN, MD
Department of General Surgery, Madigan Army Medical Center, Tacoma, Washington

NIRAV MERCHANT, BS, MS
Director, Data Science Institute, University of Arizona, Tucson, Arizona

CHRISTOPHER PRIEN, MD, MS
Research Fellow, Department of Colon and Rectal Surgery, Digestive Disease and Surgery Institute, Cleveland Clinic, Cleveland, Ohio

CAROLINE E. RICHBURG, BS
Medical Student, University of Michigan Medical School, Ann Arbor, Michigan

JOSEPH SCALEA, MD
Professor, Vice Chair of Innovation, Department of Surgery, Medical University of South Carolina, Charleston, South Carolina

ANDREW B. SCHNEIDER, MD, MSc
Department of Surgery, Assistant Professor of Surgery, The University of North Carolina at Chapel Hill, Chapel Hill, North Carolina

SHRUTHI SRINIVAS, MD
General Surgery Resident, Department of Surgery, The Ohio State University, Columbus, Ohio

MIKE WEYKAMP, MD
General Surgery Resident, Department of Surgery, University of Washington, Seattle, Washington

ANDREW J. YOUNG, MD
Assistant Professor, Division of Trauma, Critical Care, and Burn, The Ohio State University, Columbus, Ohio

Contents

The emergence of Big Data has been facilitated by technological advancements in the processing, storage, and analysis of large quantities of data. Its strength is derived from its size, ease of access, and speed of analysis, and it has enabled surgeons to investigate areas of interest that traditional research models have historically been unable to address. In the future, Big Data will likely assist in the incorporation of more advanced technologies into surgical practice, including artificial intelligence and machine learning to realize the full potential of Big Data in Surgery.

Surgical decision-making is a continuum of judgments that take place during the preoperative, intraoperative, and postoperative periods. The fundamental, and most challenging, step is determining whether a patient will benefit from an intervention given the dynamic interplay of diagnostic, temporal, environmental, patient-centric, and surgeon-centric factors. The myriad combinations of these considerations generate a wide spectrum of reasonable therapeutic approaches within the standards of care. Although surgeons may seek evidenced-based practices to support their decision-making, threats to the validity of evidence and appropriate application of evidence may influence implementation. Furthermore, a surgeon's conscious and unconscious biases may additionally determine individual practice.

The electronic medical record has fundamentally altered the way surgeons participate and practice medicine. There is now a wealth of data, once hidden behind paper records, that is, now available to surgeons to provide superior care to their patients. This article reviews the history of the electronic medical record, discusses use cases of additional data resources, and highlights the pitfalls of this relatively new technology.

Daniel Lammers and John McClellan

The practice of evidence-based medicine is the result of a multitude of research and trials aimed toward improving health-care outcomes. An understanding of the associated data remains paramount toward optimizing patient outcomes. Medical statistics commonly revolve around frequentist concepts that are convoluted and nonintuitive for nonstatisticians. Within this article, we will discuss frequentist statistics, their limitations, as well as introduce Bayesian statistics as an alternative approach for data interpretation. By doing so, we intend to highlight the importance of correct statistical interpretations through clinically relevant examples while providing a deeper understanding of the underlying philosophies of frequentist and Bayesian statistics.

Caroline E. Richburg, Lesly A. Dossett, and Tasha M. Hughes

A cognitive bias describes "shortcuts" subconsciously applied to new scenarios to simplify decision-making. Unintentional introduction of cognitive bias in surgery may result in surgical diagnostic error that leads to delayed surgical care, unnecessary procedures, intraoperative complications, and delayed recognition of postoperative complications. Data suggest that surgical error secondary to the introduction of cognitive bias results in significant harm. Thus, debiasing is a growing area of research which urges practitioners to deliberately slow decision-making to reduce the effects of cognitive bias.

Mike Weykamp and Jason Bingham

The evolution of the knowledge economy and technology industry have fundamentally changed the learning environments occupied by contemporary surgical trainees and created pressures that will force the surgical community to consider. Although some learning differences are intrinsic to the generations themselves, these differences are primarily a function of the environments in which surgeons of different generations trained. Acknowledgment of the principles of connectivism and thoughtful integration of artificial intelligence and computerized decision support tools must play a central role in charting the future course of surgical education.

Shruthi Srinivas and Andrew J. Young

Machine learning, a subtype of artificial intelligence, is an emerging field of surgical research dedicated to predictive modeling. From its inception, machine learning has been of interest in medical and surgical research. Built on traditional research metrics for optimal success, avenues of research include diagnostics, prognosis, operative timing, and surgical education, in a variety of surgical subspecialties. Machine learning represents an exciting and developing future in the world of surgical research that will not only allow for more personalized and comprehensive medical care.

Applications for artificial intelligence (AI) and machine learning in surgery include image interpretation, data summarization, automated narrative construction, trajectory and risk prediction, and operative navigation and robotics. The pace of development has been exponential, and some AI applications are working well. However, demonstrations of clinical utility, validity, and equity have lagged algorithm development and limited widespread adoption of AI into clinical practice. Outdated computing infrastructure and regulatory challenges which promote data silos are key barriers. Multidisciplinary teams will be needed to address these challenges and to build AI systems that are relevant, equitable, and dynamic.

Big Data is transforming health care. Characteristics of Big Data require data management strategies to effectively use, analyze, and apply the data. Clinicians are not typically learned in the fundamentals of these strategies which may cause a divide between collected data and data used. This article introduces the fundamentals of Big Data management and encourages clinicians to work with their information technology partners to further understand these processes and to identify opportunities for collaboration.

Data privacy in the United States is protected by a patchwork of Federal and state laws. Federal laws protect data based on the type of entity collecting and retaining the information. Unlike the European Union, there is no comprehensive privacy statute. Some statutes, such as the Health Insurance Portability and Accountability have specific requirements others like the Federal Trade Commission Act, only protect against deceptive and unfair business practices. Because of this framework, the use of personal data in the United States requires navigating through a series of complicated Federal and state statutes that are continuously being updated and amended.

The adoption of digital health services in surgical care delivery is changing the patient experience. The goal of patient-generated health data monitoring incorporated with patient-centered education and feedback is to optimally prepare patients for surgery and personalize postoperative care to improve outcomes that matter to both patients and surgeons. Challenges include the need for the adoption of new methods for implementation and evaluation and equitable application of surgical digital health interventions, with considerations for accessibility as well as the development of new diagnostics and decision support that include the needs and characteristics of all populations served.

SURGICAL CLINICS OF NORTH AMERICA

FORTHCOMING ISSUES

June 2023
Burn Management
Leopoldo C. Cancio, *Editor*

August 2023
Vascular Surgery
Ravi K. Veeraswamy and
Dawn M. Coleman, *Editors*

October 2023
Updates in Abdominal Core Health
David M. Krpata, *Editor*

RECENT ISSUES

February 2023
Breast Cancer Management
Anna Seydel and Lee G. Wilke, *Editors*

December 2022
Management of Benign Breast Disease
Melissa Kaptanian, *Editor*

October 2022
Pediatric Surgery
John Horton, *Editor*

SERIES OF RELATED INTEREST

Advances in Surgery
https://www.advancessurgery.com/
Surgical Oncology Clinics
https://www.surgonc.theclinics.com/
Thoracic Surgery Clinics
https://www.thoracic.theclinics.com/

Foreword

Surgical Clinics, Surgical Decision Making, Evidence, and Artificial Intelligence

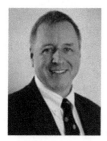

Ronald F. Martin, MD, FACS
Consulting Editor

In some respects, the beauty of being a surgeon is that one does not always have to know exactly what is actually going on, but one must always know what exactly must be done. That simple paradigm may seem simple enough at face value; it is not.

The topic of what do we know and how do we know it was the genesis of this issue of the *Surgical Clinics*. It began with a conversation that I had with one of our Guest Editors, Dr Bingham. I had just returned to Madigan Army Medical Center as a civilian surgeon years after having worked there while I was still actively in the military. The conversation wandered around several topics relating to how things have changed. One of the topics that really intrigued me in that conversation was how we were handling integrating new concepts in general. In particular, large data sets and real-time analysis and implementation. This morphed into the broader question of what we know and how do we know it is true at this time. As a result of that conversation, we set out to collect a series of ideas about what is evidence, how do we analyze it, and how do we make decisions based upon that. Dr Bingham and his co-editors, Drs Eckert and Eckert, fleshed out that list of topics and have assembled a group of people very well suited to address these questions.

While not necessarily always correct, it is extremely common to view this discussion of how we surgeons as a community gather information and put it to use, particularly as it relates to the use of technology, through a generational lens. As is mentioned in the issue, that is not always a valid construct. There are certainly members of our community that have never known the "predigital" age, but many of those whose time on Earth predates the Internet have well-developed digital skills. In fact, the entire digital age platform was developed by people who predate the "digital age."

Surg Clin N Am 103 (2023) xi–xiv
https://doi.org/10.1016/j.suc.2023.01.002
0039-6109/23/© 2023 Published by Elsevier Inc.

The development of real-time searchable digital information has been enormously useful to countless persons in all stripes of life. This utility comes with some serious caveats, however. As is described in this issue, there has been a marked expansion of sources of information for the interested person to consider in just surgery alone. I would say that in many respects this mirrors the changes in broadcast capability over the same timeframe. In the 1960s and 1970s, there were 3 major national broadcasting entities in most communities; four, once public broadcasting began its mission. The obvious downside to that framework was that those few networks essentially decided what content was relevant for all (complete with commercial biases intrinsic to the model). The upside was that most people had similar streams of information to consider and a common platform from which to discuss. For viewpoints that did not "fit well" into the mainstream networks, one had a robust print world to turn to on an individual basis. Since the advent of cable, followed by Internet, the number and variety of information sources have expanded such that is unlikely that any two people have a truly common source of input. The upside, of course, is the democratization of ideas and the ability to advance them. The downside is the democratization of ideas and the ability to advance them.

The filterless expansion of what is essentially a publishing platform (reproducing, amplifying, and transmitting information for monetary gain through subscription or advertising)—amorphous though it may be—has created an environment where all can be heard; even robots. Yet, the phenomenal increase in noise along with signal within the bandwidth does not necessarily translate into the most efficient conveyance of reliable information. While this concern is most frequently discussed today in terms of political practices, the general problem applies to the scientific community as well. We have our own share of misinformation/disinformation spread as well. Even under the most ideal circumstances, there are biases regarding the analysis of data and opinions that are permitted in the "public square" that very much limit our discussions.

One of the many byproducts of the digital age, specifically related to massively enhanced processing power, is the gathering, storage, evaluation, and distillation of large data sets. As someone who financed much of my undergraduate and medical school education by developing and writing software for various research and business purposes, I greatly appreciate the ability of computing to handle large databases. One thing I took away from that phase of my life was the need to use technology to solve the problem of my customer, as opposed to writing software that I found interesting and then have the customer find a way to use it. There is absolutely room for developing technology whose use is unclear at the moment as well. However, when it comes to real-time patient care, a certain degree of pragmatism is frequently required.

Large database analysis commonly comes up against the problem of scope. The capability to "zoom in and out" frequently changes the analysis. Missing data, variably collected data, and just plain wrong data all require analytical tools that are incompletely successful at avoiding errant conclusions. There has been a huge increase in the amount of presented and published material that is based on large data sets and analysis. I have significant concerns that much of this is not well understood by the presenters. As I have written before, when large data-based presentations are made and one asks the presenter even basic questions about how to interpret to data and/or the conclusions rendered, the stock response is, "Thank you for that excellent question. However, because our analysis is based on registry data, we do not have the granularity to address your concern." Furthermore, it not uncommon for people to present material based on data-mining for a condition that they have never ever seen or treated.

Another concern is that presentations based on large data set reviews often achieve statistical significance based on the fundamental tenets of statistics when using "large N" models. We frequently seem to forget the P value represents the likelihood that what we are seeing is the product of random chance (apologies to actual statisticians for the crudeness of the explanation), and therefore, the possibility that the correlation we infer is not accurate. Large N models frequently reduce the shape of the distribution curve and therefore reduce P value. The potential downside of that is that many large N models do not really compare things that are truly alike; as such, the actual "N" may be more elusive than one would wish. The net result of this lack of granularity and conformity of input can yield some odd results. I recall a paper that concluded that the use of antibiotics reduced length of stay for inguinal hernia repair from 14 days to 12 days. Common sense should dictate to us that any patient undergoing inguinal hernia repair in this era who had any "length of stay" beyond an outpatient procedure is already an anomaly and cannot be part of a data set to test one treatment versus another for most inguinal hernia repairs. We must understand when data analysis gives us conclusions that are incompatible with reality. In the example just given, it is fairly obvious that something is awry (other than the paper was published in the first place). In other situations, it may be far more difficult to spot an errant assessment.

For those of us who trained in surgery prior to the advent of the digital age and all its accoutrements, we have to embrace the use of data and digital options to manage our responsibilities in real time as well as educate ourselves in an efficient manner. For those who only know the Internet age, particularly those in Generation Z or I-generation, it is imperative that they also learn how to process patients in an "analog" way as well. Just as all quantum functions collapse upon observation to a single (hopefully) data point, all patients eventually narrow down to one, or at least a very small number, of surgical problems out of the universe of possibilities upon presentation. While big data is excellent at producing the list of possibilities, analog evaluation of the patient, at present, usually prevails at addressing the patient's clinical concern. And while artificial intelligence (AI) shows promise (or dread) in many areas, the reliability factor of truthfulness—either while ascertaining subtle information or relaying information—is lacking. For some time, I think the surgical world will be safe from AI replacement, although that may not last forever.

The ability to regard data and data evaluation as a platform to support understanding rather than as a final arbiter of understanding is critical. We must always interpret results in light of cumulative experience and observable facts. That said, the earth really does look flat from certain perspectives. We don't wish to reinvent the Flat Earth Society. Nor do we wish to throw away everything we think we know based on meta-analysis. Wisdom will more likely come from learning to embrace both.

To address the need to educate our younger colleagues in the art of patient "analog" care is a bit beyond the scope of this particular issue. However, I am deeply indebted to our Guest Editors, Jason Bingham, Matt Eckert, and Carly Eckert, for assembling the topics and the contributors to give each of us an excellent platform to understand how we gather, store, manage, and validate data as well as how we can use large set data analysis, machine learning, AI, and technology to maintain and improve our education and the care of our patients.

Ronald F. Martin, MD, FACS
Colonel (Retired), United States Army Reserve
Department of General Surgery
Pullman Surgical Associates
Pullman Regional Hospital and Clinic Network
825 Southeast Bishop Boulevard, Suite 130
Pullman, WA 99163, USA

E-mail address:
rfmcescna@gmail.com

Preface

Surgical Decision Making, Evidence, and Artificial Intelligence

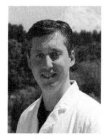
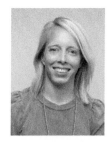
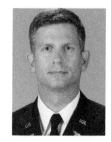

Jason Bingham, MD, FACS   Carly Eckert, MD, MPH   Matthew Eckert, MD, FACS

Editors

> *Doctors put drugs of which they know little into bodies of which they know less for diseases of which they know nothing at all.*
>
> *—Voltaire (1694-1770)*

While it is evident from this quote that Voltaire had little reverence for physicians, the modern practice of medicine would likely be unrecognizable to him. Since the days of Voltaire, evidence-based medicine (EBM), the basis of which has evolved over a century, has become the guiding principle of modern medical practice. More recently, the digital revolution has resulted in an explosion of data together with improved methods for collecting, processing, and understanding large and diverse types of data. This rapid expansion of clinical knowledge and the correspondingly ever-shortening half-life of relevant information are often expressed as an expansion of the "five V's of information" (ie, volume, velocity, variety, value, and veracity). Under this paradigm, traditional methods of data analysis and knowledge creation are simply inadequate. Thus, the next phase in the evolution of EBM will undoubtedly become more and more intertwined with emerging technologies.

In this issue of *Surgical Clinics*, we explore the impact of the digital revolution in health care and how it affects our patients. The intent of this issue is to provide a framework to understand how data are used in surgical decision making and equip surgeons with modern tools necessary to properly evaluate evidence in the era of big data. We believe that technologies such as machine learning, artificial intelligence, and computerized decision support tools have the potential to allow for more personalized, comprehensive medical care and are likely to play a central role in charting the future

Surg Clin N Am 103 (2023) xv–xvi
https://doi.org/10.1016/j.suc.2023.01.001
0039-6109/23/© 2023 Published by Elsevier Inc.

surgical.theclinics.com

of evidence-based practice. In this rapidly developing knowledge economy, it is imperative that surgeons understand, shape, and implement these advancements into their clinical practices and research.

We would like to thank Dr Ronald Martin, Consulting Editor, for providing the vision and opportunity to contribute as well as the team at Elsevier for their support and assistance in bringing this issue to completion. We are also extremely grateful to the authors for generously contributing their time and expertise. We hope this issue serves as a timely reference to how we create, manage, interpret, and apply data in the surgical care of our patients.

Jason Bingham, MD, FACS
4414 North Waterview Street
Tacoma, WA 98407, USA

Carly Eckert, MD, MPH
1023 Cleland Drive
Chapel Hill, NC 27517, USA

Matthew Eckert, MD, FACS
1023 Cleland Drive
Chapel Hill, NC 27517, USA

E-mail addresses:
jrpbingham@gmail.com (J. Bingham)
carly.m.eckert@gmail.com (C. Eckert)
matteckert1@gmail.com (M. Eckert)

Big Data in Surgery

Christopher Prien, MD, MS, Eddy P. Lincango, MD,
Stefan D. Holubar, MD, MS*

KEYWORDS

- Surgery • outcomes research • Quality • Registries • Big data
- Natural language processing • Machine learning • Artificial intelligence

KEY POINTS

- The emergence of Big Data represents the dawn of the next wave of technological advancements in surgery, which will depend on surgeons to assume a leadership role and understand, steer, and integrate these advancements into clinical practice.
- Big Data's value is inherent due to its size, ease of access, and ability to empower surgeons with clinically actionable data.
- The expanding interest in personalized health data tracking and the growing recognition of the strength of collaboratives will continue to increase the role of Big Data in clinical practice and research.

INTRODUCTION

Technology has historically helped drive improvements in medical diagnostics, therapeutics, and this has been accelerated in the digital era. In recent decades, health care has undergone a digital revolution, which has resulted in new and improved abilities to create, gather, store, analyze, and ultimately process and understand large and diverse types of electronic health information.[1] This rise of Big Data, which represents extremely large datasets often containing millions of records, and the requisite advanced analytical tools required to access and translate them into new medical knowledge, represent the next wave of advancement. For surgeons living in the information age, the ability to incorporate and use Big Data into their practices, knowingly or unknowingly, has aided in the development of personalized, patient-tailored approaches to care by allowing near instantaneous access to vast troves of information, which can help to improve surgeons' knowledge and skills.

The foundation and expansion of Big Data in current day health care was attributed to several key bureaucratic policies. Before this, in 2008, the American Medical Informatics Association recognized the need for our health-care workforce to be trained in

Department of Colon & Rectal Surgery, Digestive Disease and Surgery Institute, Cleveland Clinic, Cleveland, OH, USA
* Corresponding author. Cleveland Clinic Main Campus, 9500 Euclid Avenue. A30, Cleveland, OH 44122.
E-mail address: holubas@ccf.org

Surg Clin N Am 103 (2023) 219–232
https://doi.org/10.1016/j.suc.2022.12.002
0039-6109/23/© 2022 Elsevier Inc. All rights reserved.

surgical.theclinics.com

medical informatics and initiated the 10 × 10 (10,000 informatics trained health-care professionals by the year 2010) program (amia.org/education-events/amia-10 × 10-virtual-courses), and these programs still offer 10 × 10 Certification, now often virtually; Board certification may also be obtained in Clinical Informatics.[2]

In 2009, the United States government passed the Health Information Technology for Economic and Health (HITECH) Act (www.hipaajournal.com/what-is-the-hitech-act/), which monetarily incentivized the widespread adoption of electronic medical records, and more broadly electronic health records (EHRs).[3] With the increasing utilization of EHRs, the volume of available clinical data skyrocketed and stimulated the development of numerous clinical registries while also increasing the amount of captured clinical data, from granular discrete data such as vital signs and laboratories, to novel data such as patient-reported outcomes and measures.[3]

Subsequent to the HITECH Act, in 2012, the National Institutes of Health (NIH) accelerated the growth of Big Data in health care with the commitment of US$100 million through the Big Data to Knowledge Initiative (BD2K), which aimed to expand the footprint and utilization of Big Data (www.commonfund.nih.gov/bd2k/highlights).[4,5] Using Big Data, many surgeons hoped to address questions standard research models could not tackle with the intent of facilitating change at the clinical level in the form of improvements in health-care quality, outcomes, and patient safety while minimizing costs.[3,4]

In this article, we will define Big Data and describe the sources, value, and pitfalls of using this data to drive clinical research while also highlighting some of the ways it has already affected current surgical practice and what can be expected moving into the future.

What is "Big Data"?

The term "Big Data" logically will make one think of very big numbers or large sets of data. Big Data is used to describe large collections of structured, semistructured, or unstructured data, which grow exponentially over time. Structured data is highly formatted and structured, typically defined by a data-dictionary and is quantitative in the form of values or numbers. An example of semistructured data is clinic notes that contain both discrete elements and free text. Unstructured data has no predefined format or organization and may be qualitative in the form of free text operative reports and multimedia such as photos and video.

Given the size and complexity of Big Data, full understanding of many Big Data datasets is beyond human comprehension, thus traditional biostatical applications, procedures, and systems used to process and analyze data may be ineffective and require "basic" artificial intelligence (AI) interfaces such as natural language processing (NLP) and machine-learning, which can be used or taught to "read" free-text or images to abstract and translate the data into more convenient, interpretable "chunks" of data.[6,7]

There have been several attempts to pragmatically define the term Big Data. In 2001, Doug Laney first defined "Big Data" using the 3Vs: Volume, Velocity, and Variety in that it represented extremely large volumes of data acquired rapidly from heterogenous sources.[8] This has been expanded to the 5 Vs, 7 Vs, and more recently the 17Vs (**Table 1**).[9] When the BDKI was passed, it had a more formal definition of Big Data consisting of (1) a small number of groups producing very large amounts of data as part of specifically funded projects to (voluntarily) produce resources for the entire research community, (2) individual investigators producing large datasets empowered by the use of readily available new technologies, and (3) numerous sources that each produce small datasets whose value is amplified by aggregating or integrating with other data.[4]

Table 1 The "17 Vs" of big data		
# Data Characteristic	Data Attribute/Synonym	Description
1 Volume	Size of data	Quantity of collected/stored data
2 Velocity	Speed of data	Transfer rate between source and end-user
3 Value	Importance of data	Business value
4 Variety	Type of data	Text, images, audio/video
5 Veracity	Quality of data	*"Garbage in*, garbage out"
6 Validity	Authenticity of data	Translatable into useable information
7 Volatility	Longevity of data	Duration of usefulness; how long is the data useful
8 Visualization	Representation of the data	Conversion of data into an (abstract) mental image
9 Virality	Spreading speed of data	Dissemination rate to individual users
10 Viscosity	Lag of data	Difference between when data occurred and was recorded
11 Variability	Differentiation of data	Ability to efficiently differentiate between signal and noise
12 Venue	Location/platform of data	Different sources/systems (ie, local/ private vs cloud/public)
13 Vocabulary	Terminology of data	Data model, structure, dictionary
14 Vagueness	Indistinctness of data	Is the data meaningful?
15 Verbosity	Amalgamation of different datum	The redundancy of the information available at different sources
16 Voluntariness	Ability of the data to help	Willful availability
17 Versatility	Adaptability of data	Flexibility to be used differently/in different contexts
– Complexity	Correlation of data	Inconsistencies in data format or structure when merging data

Adapted from Panimalar A, Shree V, Kathrine V. The 17 V's Of Big Data. International Research Journal of Engineering and Technology. Sep 2017;4(9):329-333

Practically speaking, for surgeons, Big Data is best understood as the amalgamation of an abundance of data sources along the patient care path, often including both administrative and clinical data points, to create a rich, comprehensive, and clinically relevant dataset.[10] The dataset is then analyzed to help drive improvements in patient care, via quality improvement (QI) needs or clinical research questions. An example of Big Data most readers will be familiar with is the American College of Surgeons-National Quality Improvement Program (ACS-NSQIP). What readers may not realize is that NSQIP, during the 15-year period from 2005 to 2020, with greater than 700 international contributing hospitals with upward of 300 variables per case, as of 2020 has accumulated 7,886,515 surgical cases or greater than 2 billion discrete data points (www.facs.org/quality-programs/data-and-registries/acs-nsqip/participant-use-data-file/).

As stated previously, technological advancements and the development of tools capable of recording digital data (often remotely) fostered improvements in the capacity to store, process, and share via networking large swaths of data.[11] Due to advancements in semiconductor computer chip technology, and consistent with Moore's Law that states the number of components per integrated circuit chip (and computer speed/storage capacity) doubles every 18 months. Current personal computers and laptops now have the computational abilities previously only available on supercomputers, whereas cloud computing has allowed essentially limitless storage capacity. Resultantly, it has become possible to create enormous, readily available, and accessible datasets of digital information, often without a clearly defined, unified purpose when initially collected.[10,11]

These datasets are categorized as either clinical or administrative, with administrative data becoming increasingly used to evaluate surgical outcomes and audit surgical quality.[12] The conduct of Big Data research is therefore reliant on a surgeon or researcher's ability to analyze these datasets to determine what hypotheses can be answered from the available data, a fundamental difference from traditional observational research study design.[4] However, analyzing these massive, complex datasets can lead to valuable insights, which would not have been obtainable through analysis of smaller data pools.[3] As this style of research continues to evolve, researchers must remain wary of the strengths and weaknesses associated with these approaches.[6]

Sources of Big Data

In most cases, the primary data source for populating large clinical and administrative databases is the EHR. The expansion of EHR usage established the foundation for Big Data because it consolidated patient data into centralized access points that could be easily queried either by staff to extract points of interest or by specialized software capable of quickly screening thousands of records and extracting needed data. The significance of EHRs is more detailed in the article "Clinical Informatics and the Electronic Medical Record". However, it is likely as health care becomes increasingly digital that any level of interaction capable of generating patient-specific data could be used as a source. This, in theory, will include personal, mobile health hardware and software applications, such as smartwatches and smart rings in line with the "quantified self" phenomenon. As these approaches become increasingly used, it will represent an expanded source of data, one with a level of granularity previously unmatched especially because it refers to health as opposed to illness.

When it comes to data utilization, databases represent the primary form of data repository, which may then be accessed by surgeons, clinical researchers, data scientists, and their support staff. When determining which database to use, it remains critical to have a firm understanding of what kind of data is stored in the database and the source of that data. As of 2014, there were greater than 120 clinical data registries being used in the United States.[3] These included a combination of large single-institution registries, such as The Cleveland Clinic Ileoanal Pouch Registry, which contains clinical long-term outcomes and patient reported outcomes (PROs) on greater than 6000 pouch patients, as well as (inter)national level, multi-institutional databases such as ACS-NSQIP. **Table 2** lists some of the most common national registries and databases.

In many respects, the development of large databases such as the ACS-NSQIP (www.facs.org/quality-programs/data-and-registries/acs-nsqip/), the National Inpatient Sample (NIS)HYPERLINK "http://www.hcup-us.ahrq.gov/nisoverview.jsp" \o "http://www.hcup-us.ahrq.gov/nisoverview.jsp"www.hcup-us.ahrq.gov/nisoverview.jsp, and the Metabolic and Bariatric Surgery Accreditation and Quality Improvement Program (MBSQAIP; www.facs.org/quality-programs/accreditation-and-verification/metabolic-and-bariatric-surgery-accreditation-and-quality-improvement-program/) signified the dawn of the Big Data era in surgery.[11] It is anticipated that as Big Data

Table 2
List of some of the major databases and registries used in surgical research

Clinical Databases	Administrative Databases
National Surgical Quality Program (NSQIP)	Center for Medicare and Medicaid Services
Society of Thoracic Surgeons National Database	Healthcare Cost and Utilization Project National Inpatient Sample
Multicenter Perioperative Outcomes Group	Humana administrative claims database
Anesthesia Quality Institute's National Anesthesia Clinical Outcomes Registry	Medicaid Statistical Information System
American College of Surgeons National Trauma Databank	Children's Health Insurance Program
National Cancer Database	
Surveillance, Epidemiology, and End Results	
Metabolic and Bariatric Surgery Accreditation and Quality Improvement Program	
NSQIP – Inflammatory Bowel Disease Collaborative	

utilization continues to expand, database architecture will continue to evolve with new models developed to refine and streamline surgeon access and usage.[13]

SHIFTING THE RESEARCH PARADIGM

In the current era of evidence-based medicine (EBM), the randomized controlled trial (RCT) remains the gold standard research model. By far the most valuable aspect of an RCT is its ability to directly compare interventions while balancing and controlling for known and unknown confounders and reducing bias through randomization, and providing insights into, not proof of, causality.[14] Historically, this approach has been used by surgeons to establish efficacy of surgical procedures and obtain optimal patient outcomes. However, in surgery, RCTs are difficult to conduct and may be ladened with challenges such as poor accrual, limited generalizability, copious resource utilization (ie, time, costs), and biased results.[14]

Big Data research presents itself as a new alternative, which does not attempt to replace RCTs but rather aims to enhance study design, improve conductance, and overcome limitations.[14,15] The benefits of Big Data research are inherent in its accessibility (ie, the Framingham heart study), relatively limited cost to individual investigators, ability to power studies to detect even minor differences, amass rare cases, generalizability of findings, and the ability to address questions not feasible for an RCT to answer due to either complexity, cost, or ethical impediments.[4,14–17] Furthermore, Big Data can be used to supplement RCTs by helping to inform pretrial power calculations and conferring posttrial external validation.[14,16] However, Big Data research also has its own limitations, including coding errors, missing data, and the determination of clinical significance, various biases, and societal costs, all points which prevent more widespread utilization.

The Value of Big Data

In general, Big Data enables studies to be performed faster and cheaper than traditional study designs, with minimal risk to patients.[16] This extends from the fact that after creation of a registry or database, the data is continuously updated and available for analysis. There is no need for meticulous chart review or subject recruitment with each new study. In eliminating the need for researchers to perform data collection, time and energy can be reappropriated toward hypothesis-generation and data analysis. This is in stark contrast to traditional study designs, which at times requires months or years for grant writing and seeking, and then adequate number of subjects to be recruited, inclusion and exclusion notwithstanding. As a result, Big Data studies cost far less to conduct, although one must acknowledge there is cost associated with registry maintenance and employment of a database manager. For example, NSQIP requires an annual subscription fee of approximately US$30,000, as well as a full-time surgical clinical reviewer registered nurse salary of roughly US$80,000 per year.

In addition to the practical aspects of Big Data, another major benefit is the inherent strength of the data itself. Many times, databases contain data derived from multiple institutions, and using such large data can help researchers increase the power of their studies and permit them to conduct more sophisticated analyses.[16] However, Big Data does not always equate to high-quality data or, more importantly, a quality study. Therefore, it remains paramount for researchers to carefully design their study based on a narrowed, specific research question and focused hypothesis, with the chosen data source limitations in mind.[16]

In a sense, Big Data represents a new level of knowledge and ultimately wisdom: "Information is power."[13] Historically medical research has been limited by traditional study designs because it was impossible to accrue an adequate number of subjects to study topics such as rare diseases or make accurate evaluations about rare, single-digit outcomes such as anastomotic leak or venous thromboembolism (VTE).[15] Big Data addresses this issue. However, when thinking about the evaluation of surgical outcomes, it is important to recall that statistical significance does not always equate to clinical significance. Large datasets may be overpowered especially about continuous variables, such that a small difference in age or specific laboratory values among groups may be highly statistically different, yet clinically irrelevant. Therefore, surgeons must play a vital role in interpreting study results within an appropriate clinical context as well as aid in translating results into meaningful clinical change.[12]

The most common types of research performed using Big Data are comparative case-control and retrospective cohort studies (aka descriptive case series). Once a question is developed, data can be queried for the points of interest with relative ease. This can be especially useful for surgeons seeking to identify modifiable versus nonmodifiable risk factors, and rare disease/events/outcomes.[15] In a recent review by Zhu and colleagues, the authors noted that Big Data could be instrumental in altering the practice of plastic surgery by helping to identify risk factors and types of procedures that result in worse outcomes.[4] Although typically the results of retrospective studies are considered inferior to their prospective counterparts, Big Data can help provide an element of strong external validation, as well as sheer number of cases.[11] Furthermore, when studying a topic in which an RCT is not ethically or financially feasible, Big Data is capable of providing quality information to advance surgical knowledge in a manner single-center series are unable to.[11] In another example, modern networked meta-analysis would not be possible without the National Library of Medicine's PubMed interface to more than 34 million citations (https://pubmed.ncbi.nlm.nih.gov/about/) and other repositories that are Big Data sources themselves.

Another area where Big Data analysis has proved useful is in evaluation of healthcare systems because it enables assessment of processes with respect to costs and outcomes. This is particularly true of administrative databases. Targarona *and colleagues* discussed the role of Big Data in the development of *"Business*

Intelligence" and how surgeons should use data to identify potential areas of resource utilization, which may benefit from more efficient management and optimization.[13] Many systems in the United States have instituted Big Data for this purpose to increase efficiency and minimize losses by developing administrative and clinical dashboards, especially in the setting of the COVID-19 pandemic. However, thinking more broadly; it may be that Big Data's role should be even greater as some authors see potential for Big Data to help provide rationale for decisions regarding health-care policy.[15] This would require a wider acceptance of Big Data analytics, as well as careful, expert understanding and interpretation of findings.

One of the more valuable ways by which Big Data has been used is in the reform of quality assessment and benchmarks. Before the creation of large surgical registries and databases, surgeons relied on comparison of quality metrics among individual practices or within individual health-care systems. Databases such as NSQIP and NIS have provided regulatory bodies with a means to create a system of nationwide benchmarking, comparing patient outcomes on a nationwide scale, which has been useful in assessing regional and institutional performance as well as modification of outcome-based reimbursements and payments.[13] Surgeon application of findings extracted from Big Data studies has also helped further drive the concept of "Precision Medicine," in which large volumes of data have been effective at guiding medical decision-making at a high level with a degree of precision previously unattainable.[13]

The potential benefits of Big Data remain vast, and the excitement around it stems from the way it has helped advance medicine, although its usage and application remain relatively limited. It is easy to fathom the breadth of impact Big Data can have, stretching from technological improvements and better predictive models and algorithms to better, more safely controlled implementation of medical devices, to optimization of decision-making, payments, and cost reductions.[13] These include simple decision-support tools such as best practice alert pop-ups, real-time risk stratification, and early-warning systems. However, before arriving at these downstream benefits of Big Data utilization, it remains important to understand how studies using Big Data differ from traditional studies as well as how surgeons can arrive at findings capable of implementation into practice.

Pitfalls of Big Data

Some of the greatest resistance to Big Data extends from concerns over the data quality and, ultimately, the clinical significance of Big Data study findings. When databases and registries first arose, there was no standardized creation process. Initially, single-center sources were often the most comprehensive and detailed as centers prided themselves on meticulous data collection but these processes were often noted to degrade over time with staff turnover. In contrast, larger, multicenter registries often had a great deal of heterogeneity with respect to data quality and density.[15] Furthermore, in many cases, big databases were frequently noted to have errors, missing data, and a lack of organization, which ultimately lessened the strength, reliability, and consolidation of the data.[11,17,18]

In 2015, Nouraei *and colleagues* confirmed these concerns when they evaluated the reliability of surgical clinical coding and administrative databases and found that in many cases (51%) initial coding was inaccurate and required modification.[19] The authors concluded that not only was surgical coding prone to subjectivity, variability, and error but that understanding the variability of informatics is crucial to ultimately determining the clinical applicability of administrative data in surgical outcomes improvement. Bedard and colleagues further highlighted the variability of big database data with their study, which compared total hip arthroplasty (THA) 30-day outcomes

reported by the NSQIP, NIS, Medicare Claims (MED) Standard Analytical Files (www.
cms.gov/Research-Statistics-Data-and-Systems/Files-for-Order/LimitedDataSets/
StandardAnalyticalFiles) databases.[20] The authors found considerable variability in
THA complication rates depending on the database used and highlighted the importance for researchers to understand how data is extracted, who is extracting the data,
and what the database intention is, so as to pick the data source best suited to answer
their question. For NSQIP and NIS, the problem with validity has been addressed via
the use of training, extensive supporting documentation, and random auditing for
quality-assurance.

Aside from the question surrounding data validity, the other major issue with Big
Data was translating the information into clinically relevant action.[3] Many surgeons
and researchers recognized the benefits of having large data sets that could be
quickly analyzed by statistical programs; however, they noted that a well-developed
hypothesis and research question remained paramount because the high power
generated by these databases often resulted in studies reporting statistically significant findings for the sake of publication without any clinical premise, a process referring to as "fishing expeditions" and often are not practice changing by any
means.[4,12,16] Some authors have also pointed out that Big Data upends traditional
research methodology because it may provide all the data before a hypothesis is
generated or a study is designed to address the hypothesis; with Big Data, researchers must figure out what questions may be asked of the data and avoid fishing
expedition type approaches.[6]

The tendency of Big Data analyses to be overpowered is mentioned above. Other
areas of consideration pertain to the ethics and legal considerations surrounding
Big Data, which are further explained in article: "Data Sharing, Privacy, and Legal
Considerations".

Lyu *and colleagues* highlighted the difficulty in performing clinically relevant
research in their review, which described how difficult it was to perform sarcoma
research using Big Data because databases lacked clinically relevant architecture
and disease-specific data points; they emphasized that disease-specific databases
may become more valuable.[8] The NSQIP Inflammatory Bowel Disease (IBD) Collaborative recognized this limitation as the first disease-specific NSQIP module. This
collaboration was formed in 2017 with the intent of improving surgical practice for patients with IBD by evaluating outcomes across major US centers.[21,22] To date, we
have implemented 17 disease-specific variables including details on indications, bio-
logics, techniques, and VTE location and prophylaxis data from 23 IBD centers of
excellence and is an excellent example of a national collaborative, which started as
a grass-roots effort.

The Power of Collaboratives

A key aspect required for the next step in the evolution of Big Data is the cultivation
and expansion of multi-institutional collaboratives. Breaking away from the traditional
model of single-center data silos limited by institutional exposure, collaboratives enables the development of robust databases and evolution of the current data system.[8]
However, this process requires extensive, multidisciplinary efforts from policy makers,
stakeholders, and data scientists with surgeons taking up the mantle of leadership.[8]
Ultimately, surgeons must recognize and participate in the expansion of the data
ecosystem with the aim of optimizing the processes of data inflow and outflow to
maximize clinical applicability.[3] There have been several examples of the power of collaboratives in surgery, including the NSQIP IBD Collaborative mentioned above.

One of the largest and most important collaboratives of all time is the GlobalSurg collaborative (www.globalsurgeryunit.org/) funded by the British National Institute for Health and Care Research. They believe in fostering national and international research networks to improve surgical outcomes. Their latest project, COVIDSurg, was a global effort aimed at examining the impact of the COVID-19 pandemic across numerous fields of surgery. More than 20 articles have been published since its inception, and the collaborative received a Guinness World Record for the most authors on a single peer-reviewed academic article with more than 15,025 collaborators from across 116 countries (www.guinnessworldrecords.com/world-records/653537-most-authors-on-a-single-peer-reviewed-academic-paper).[23–26] One of the authors of this article (E.P.L.) played a leading role in the COVIDSurg project.

As more collaborations are formed and the surgical data ecosystem evolves, the knowledge gained from analyzing Big Data will undoubtedly lead to revolutions in clinical practice.

How has Big Data Influenced Surgery?

Although we are currently living at the tip of the iceberg of Big Data in surgery, some authors have already illustrated its positive impact. Research themes have ranged from access to surgery and surgical outcomes to patient expenditure and genomic studies.[10,27] This data has driven QI processes and helped significantly influence clinical practice. One prime example of this is the Surveillance, Epidemiology, and End Results database, which has shaped the management of colorectal cancer because numerous studies have been published using its national data.

Another example of Big Data's positive influence was described by Depypere *and colleagues* in their study on the use of deep inferior epigastric perforator free flaps for breast reconstruction.[17] In their article, the investigators identified anemia and *low postoperative mean arterial pressure* as significant risk factors associated with the need for revisional surgery. The authors concluded their findings were only possible through the analysis of Big Data, which provided them with sufficient power to assess these factors, and they highlighted how traditionally suspected risk factors, such as anesthesia time, were not found to be significant when analyzed on a broader scale. Although, Depypere and his team did caution readers that association does not necessarily indicate causation, an important distinction to recall when conducting clinical research.

In 2019, Maguire and colleagues used the National Cancer Database to study a rare disease, primary colonic lymphoma.[28] The goal of this study was to evaluate the short-term and long-term outcomes of 2153 patients with primary colonic lymphoma who underwent nonpalliative surgery so as to inform treatment decisions and improve patient counseling. Their research found 30-day and 90-day mortality rates of 5.6% and 11.1%, respectively, that many patients did not achieve an R0 resection (46%), and only 39% of patients received adjuvant chemotherapy despite its favorable association with improved overall survival. Although this study underscored the unfavorable realities of patients undergoing surgery for primary colonic lymphoma, it also highlighted the ability of Big Data to depict the heterogeneity of care provided to patients with rare diseases and the need for standardization of treatment strategies with the goal of improving patient-centered outcomes. Srinivas *and colleagues* used a Big Data approach to predictive analytics with respect to renal transplantation. The authors noted that analysis of Big Data allowed for more efficacious prediction models of graft loss and mortality because of the size of the data points included and furthermore was a clinically relevant point, which could be used to optimize patient outcomes.[29]

With respect to advancing collaboratives, since the inception of the GlobalSurg collaborative, COVID-19 guidelines on the timing of elective surgery in England and Spain have been updated.[30,31] These reports have triggered the development of an extensive and important QI program in England. This initiative aims at avoiding unnecessary long waiting lists for elective procedures and surgery due to the COVID-19 pandemic, ultimately, enhancing the management of preventable and treatable diseases (eg, colonoscopy for colorectal cancer screening).

Big Data has also played a role in advancing technology for surgeons and endoscopists. The software behind endoscopic technologies has begun incorporating Big Data analytics resulting in the ability to generate patient-specific models that help guide navigation and procedural planning.[32] Taken one step further, this same analytics capability has also been incorporated with AI during colonoscopy to help identify colonic polyps and predict likelihood of malignancy in vivo.[33] The ability to model and construct 3D imagery and visualization is paramount to robotic surgery to assemble the operative imagery and track robotic instruments intra-abdominally.[32] These exciting technological advancements have only been possible due to the incorporation systems and software capable of processing massive amounts of data in a near real-time fashion.

Although more widespread use of Big Data is at an inflection point, it is worth noting that most of the studies have been performed in high-income countries with the capabilities to gather reliable data. The participation of low-income and middle-income countries in Big Data projects is limited, and the impact of Big Data in these countries remains to be elucidated and represents another frontier for Big Data analytics.[10,34]

How to Improve Big Data?

With the continued expansion and incorporation of Big Data into surgical research and practice, improvements to its usage and structure will help facilitate broader acceptance and application. One of the most obvious ways to improve the usage of Big Data is to train surgeons on how to properly use this data when conducting studies. The first step to this is educating surgeons on what types of queries Big Data may be useful in answering and how to construct a hypothesis or question that Big Data can answer.[35–37] In creating a very narrowed, specific question, the available data can then be queried for specific data points and helps avoid getting bogged down in excessive amounts of irrelevant data. However, in addition to training researchers to ask the right questions and obtain the correct data, there remains a need for an overhaul of traditional statistical education because Big Data requires different statistical approaches to analysis by approaches such as the 10 × 10 Clinical Informatics program mentioned above.[38] At the end of this all, it remains critical to then be able to represent the data in a meaningful manner visually and determine logical conclusions. Keeping in mind that the goal is to identify points that can drive actionable clinical change.

Another means to broaden the utilization of Big Data is by improving the reliability and ease of obtaining the data. At a basic level, creating databases to prioritize clinically relevant points and shifting toward more disease-specific databases will likely result in more focused and accessible data. Creating training programs and common language for coders would help minimize some of the subjectivity and errors associated with data extraction. Streamlining and automating the data extraction process by use of formatted templates and operative notes would help further minimize errors and duplications while also eliminating the most time-consuming aspect of Big Data studies.[1,17] NLP, as mentioned, is a form of AI that provides computers with the ability to "read" text, spoken words, or images. Its application in Big Data is one that makes researchers capable of querying and indexing large volumes of medical records for "keywords" or key features and then producing quantifiable and useable data. In fact, multiple studies examining the accuracy and effectiveness of NLP compared with traditional data extraction methods have demonstrated NLP's superiority, especially concerning surgical outcomes.[39,40] In addition, the limitations of these approaches may be partially overcome by the sheer volume of data NLP can access and report on.

The continued expansion and incorporation of Big Data will continue to drive further technological and computing advancements; however, the incorporation of additional elements of AI including machine learning will catapult Big Data to another level.[13] Although some surgeons have recognized this, it is also acknowledged that the groundwork and a firm understanding of how to maximize the clinical benefits of this type of research is required to fully maximize the technology.[41] Surgeons are positioned to integrate more AI elements with the potential benefits include improvement in patient outcomes, streamlining of physician workflow, and revelation of novel associations.[41,42] However, this may require further database optimization to make them less heterogenous and incompatible. Furthermore, because the data become more widely used and incorporated into clinical practice, the health-care system will likely need to institute modern quality requirements, database compatibility criteria to facilitate data pooling, and improve data governance for access and distribution standards, an element for which block chain may offer a solution.[10,43] More detail on the applicability of Big Data in machine learning and AI is found in article: "Interpretation and Use of Applied/Operational Machine Learning and Artificial Intelligence in Surgery".

FUTURE DIRECTIONS FOR THE USE OF BIG DATA IN SURGERY

Big data is in an early stage of development but its horizon is promising. Translating data into action is the biggest challenge. The current focus on surgery outcomes is shifting to include data on activities of daily living and genomics.[27] This panorama is supported by the increased use of smart gadgets that enables the amalgamation of information from multiple sources on an individual level.[44] Moreover, funding institutions are encouraging the evolution of new technologies in Big Data (eg, NIH grants, grants.nih.gov/grants/guide/pa-files/PA-14-154.html) and the new AI algorithms are speeding up the statistical analysis of large databases, which is discussed more in detail in the article "Interpretation and Use of Applied/Operational Machine Learning and Artificial Intelligence in Surgery".

Finally, some authors have suggested that as the role of Big Data in surgery continues to expand, patients will be able to use the data to be educated on surgical procedures, outcomes, and means by which they can modify risk factors to improve outcomes by using perioperative "Avatar" constructs.[45] However, to get to this point, there remains a need to create applications and data outflows such that specific moments in clinical care can be identified as optimal for data collection and the results of analysis can be applied.[3] The penultimate goal is to create a system in which patient-level data collection is automated and streamlined at such a level as to provide surgeons with real-time, actionable data that can be used to impact patient care before or as it occurs.[29]

The future of Big Data is both promising and exciting. As surgeons, we will be required to broaden our abilities to fully maximize the benefits Big Data will provide. The continued interweaving of Big Data into daily practice will require surgeons to become clinical informaticians in such that it will be necessary to be able to routinely collect, decipher, analyze, and integrate Big Data findings into changes in clinical practice.[1] In theory, a surgeon's ability to obtain and synthesize information from various sources and settings to make clinical decisions makes them well prepared for this future role.[1] However, at this time, most surgeons are underrepresented in this role but remain paramount to determine the best means to effectively create and implement health information technologies into surgical practice.[1]

DISCLOSURE

S D. Holubar Shionogi and Takeda consultant fees.

CLINICS CARE POINTS

- Big Data studies have been vital in studying the surgical outcomes of patients with rare diseases such as colonic lymphoma and emphasizing the need to establish standardized treatment strategies.
- The growing use of smart gadgets to track and collect granular, patient-level data likely represents the next major source of Big Data; creating a process to streamline the collection and analysis of this information remains the key to unlocking its ability to make real-time impacts on patient care.
- Big Data utilization has enabled the development and advancement of surgical technologies as evidenced by robotic surgery platforms and the incorporation of AI in endoscopic software, which has translated to enhanced prevention and management of a spectrum of diseases.

REFERENCES

1. Zhao J, Forsythe R, Langerman A, et al. The value of the surgeon informatician. J Surg Res 2020;252:264–71.
2. Feldman SS, Hersh W. Evaluating the AMIA-OHSU 10x10 program to train healthcare professionals in medical informatics. AMIA Annu Symp Proc 2008;2008: 182–6.
3. Coffron M, Opelka F. Big promise and big challenges for big heath care data. Bull Am Coll Surg 2015;100(4):10–6.
4. Zhu VZ, Tuggle CT, Au AF. Promise and limitations of big data research in plastic surgery. Ann Plast Surg 2016;76(4):453–8.
5. Margolis R, Derr L, Dunn M, et al. the national institutes of health's big data to knowledge (BD2K) initiative: capitalizing on biomedical big data. J Am Med Inform Assoc 2014;21(6):957–8.
6. Burke JP. Data, data everywhere, and not a spot to think. Colorectal Dis 2018; 20(11):953–4.
7. Chen M, Mao S, Liu Y. Big data: a survey. Mobile NetwAppl 2014;19:171–209.
8. Lyu HG, Haider AH, Landman AB, et al. The opportunities and shortcomings of using big data and national databases for sarcoma research. Cancer 2019; 125(17):2926–34.
9. Panimalar A, Shree V, Kathrine V. The 17 V's of big data. Int Res J Eng Technology 2017;4(9):329–33.
10. Knight SR, Ots R, Maimbo M, et al. Systematic review of the use of big data to improve surgery in low- and middle-income countries. Br J Surg 2019;106(2): e62–72.
11. Balla A, Batista Rodriguez G, Corradetti S, et al. Outcomes after bariatric surgery according to large databases: a systematic review. Langenbecks Arch Surg 2017;402(6):885–99.

12. Hong MK, Skandarajah AR, Hayes IP. Administrative data: what surgeons should know about big data. ANZ J Surg 2017;87(9):650–1.
13. Targarona EM, Balla A, Batista G. Big data and surgery: the digital revolution continues. Cir Esp (Engl Ed 2018;96(5):247–9. Big data y cirugia: la revolucion digital continua.
14. de Geus SWL, Sachs TE, Tseng JF. Big data vs. clinical trials in HPB surgery. J Gastrointest Surg 2020;24(5):1127–37.
15. Sessler DI. Big Data-and its contributions to peri-operative medicine. Anaesthesia 2014;69(2):100–5.
16. Massie AB, Kucirka LM, Segev DL. Big data in organ transplantation: registries and administrative claims. Am J Transpl 2014;14(8):1723–30.
17. Depypere B, Herregods S, Denolf J, et al. 20 years of DIEAP flap breast reconstruction: a big data analysis. Sci Rep 2019;9(1):12899.
18. Murthy SC. Big Data... Small Conclusion Chest 2020;157(5):1060–1.
19. Nouraei SA, Hudovsky A, Frampton AE, et al. A Study of clinical coding accuracy in surgery: implications for the use of administrative big data for outcomes management. Ann Surg 2015;261(6):1096–107.
20. Bedard NA, Pugely AJ, McHugh MA, et al. Big data and total hip arthroplasty: how do large databases compare? J Arthroplasty 2018;33(1):41–45 e3.
21. Eisenstein S, Holubar SD, Hilbert N, et al. The ACS national surgical quality improvement program-inflammatory bowel disease collaborative: design, implementation, and validation of a disease-specific module. Inflamm Bowel Dis 2019; 25(11):1731–9.
22. Luo WY, Holubar SD, Bordeianou L, et al. Better characterization of operation for ulcerative colitis through the National surgical quality improvement program: A 2-year audit of NSQIP-IBD. Am J Surg 2021;221(1):174–82.
23. Collaborative CO. Mortality and pulmonary complications in emergency general surgery patients with COVID-19: A large international multicenter study. J Trauma Acute Care Surg 2022;93(1):59–65.
24. Collaborative CO. Outcomes and their state-level variation in patients undergoing surgery with perioperative SARS-CoV-2 infection in the USA: a prospective multicenter study. Ann Surg 2022;275(2):247–51.
25. Collaborative CO, GlobalSurg C. Timing of surgery following SARS-CoV-2 infection: an international prospective cohort study. Anaesthesia 2021;76(6):748–58.
26. Collaborative CO, GlobalSurg C. Effects of pre-operative isolation on postoperative pulmonary complications after elective surgery: an international prospective cohort study. Anaesthesia 2021;76(11):1454–64.
27. Cuenca AG, Gentile LF, Lopez MC, et al. Development of a genomic metric that can be rapidly used to predict clinical outcome in severely injured trauma patients. Crit Care Med 2013;41(5):1175–85.
28. Maguire LH, Geiger TM, Hardiman KM, et al. Surgical management of primary colonic lymphoma: Big data for a rare problem. J Surg Oncol 2019;120(3):431–7.
29. Srinivas TR, Taber DJ, Su Z, et al. Big data, predictive analytics, and quality improvement in kidney transplantation: a proof of concept. Am J Transpl 2017; 17(3):671–81.
30. El-Boghdadly K, Cook TM, Goodacre T, et al. Timing of elective surgery and risk assessment after SARS-CoV-2 infection: an update: A multidisciplinary consensus statement on behalf of the Association of Anaesthetists, Centre for Perioperative Care, Federation of Surgical Specialty Associations, Royal College of Anaesthetists, Royal College of Surgeons of England. Anaesthesia 2022;77(5): 580–7.

31. Morales-Garcia D, Docobo-Durantez F, Capitan Vallvey JM, et al. Consensus of the ambulatory surgery commite section of the Spanish Association of Surgeons on the role of ambulatory surgery in the SARS-CoV-2 pandemic. Cir Esp (Engl Ed 2022;100(3):115–24.
32. Luo X, Mori K, Peters TM. advanced endoscopic navigation: surgical big data, methodology, and applications. Annu Rev Biomed Eng 2018;20:221–51.
33. Antonelli G, Gkolfakis P, Tziatzios G, et al. Artificial intelligence-aided colonoscopy: Recent developments and future perspectives. World J Gastroenterol 2020;26(47):7436–43.
34. Nepogodiev D, Covidsurg, GlobalSurg C. Timing of surgery following SARS-CoV-2 infection: country income analysis. Anaesthesia 2022;77(1):111–2.
35. Schultze JL. Teaching 'big data' analysis to young immunologists. Nat Immunol 2015;16(9):902–5.
36. Au-Yong-Oliveira M, Pesqueira A, Sousa MJ, et al. the potential of big data research in healthcare for medical doctors' learning. J Med Syst 2021;45(1):13.
37. Syzdykova A, Malta A, Zolfo M, et al. Open-source electronic health record systems for low-resource settings: systematic review. JMIR Med Inform 2017; 5(4):e44.
38. Weissgerber TL. Learning from the past to develop data analysis curricula for the future. Plos Biol 2021;19(7):e3001343.
39. Mellia JA, Basta MN, Toyoda Y, et al. natural language processing in surgery: a systematic review and meta-analysis. Ann Surg 2021;273(5):900–8.
40. Thirukumaran CP, Zaman A, Rubery PT, et al. natural language processing for the identification of surgical site infections in orthopaedics. J Bone Joint Surg Am 2019;101(24):2167–74.
41. Cobb AN, Benjamin AJ, Huang ES, et al. Big data: More than big data sets. Surgery 2018;164(4):640–2.
42. Hashimoto DA, Rosman G, Rus D, et al. artificial intelligence in surgery: promises and perils. Ann Surg 2018;268(1):70–6.
43. Dhindsa K, Bhandari M, Sonnadara RR. What's holding up the big data revolution in healthcare? BMJ 2018;363:k5357.
44. Murdoch TB, Detsky AS. The inevitable application of big data to health care. JAMA 2013;309(13):1351–2.
45. Lister C, Davies M. Big Data–of the people, for the people, by the people. Anaesthesia 2014;69(5):513–4.

Categories of Evidence and Methods in Surgical Decision-Making

Samuel P. Carmichael II, MD, MS[a],*, David M. Kline, PhD[b]

KEYWORDS

- Surgical decision-making • Levels of evidence • Risk assessment
- Evidence-based practice

KEY POINTS

- Surgical decision-making requires integration of multiple objective and subjective pieces of evidence/inputs.
- Objective evidence in the surgical literature can be confounded by multiple biases.
- Recognizing these biases within the surgical literature is essential to categorizing evidence and developing a reliable fund of knowledge.

INTRODUCTION

Scientific investigation is fundamentally an effort to establish relationships between cause and effect. Like human interactions within a society, scientific relationships provide a model through which we interpret disease and treatment. Such models are both complex and iterative, and our attempts to understand the world around us are subject to multiple confounders and biases. As a result, the journey to derive truth in light of these cognitive fragilities has taken multiple millennia. Even at present, we have relatively few cures to alleviate human suffering. Nonetheless, our capacity for treatment discovery is heavily influenced by our ability to uncover the correct causal model. It is therefore imperative for each generation of surgeons to systematically evaluate current practices and question their incongruences.

Washington on His Deathbed (**Fig. 1**) by Junius Stearns reveals the bedside scene of a dying president. Following his Farewell Address in 1796, George Washington retired to his Mount Vernon estate, south of what is present-day Washington DC, at the age of

[a] Department of Surgery, Wake Forest School of Medicine, Medical Center Boulevard, Winston-Salem, NC 27157, USA; [b] Division of Public Health Sciences, Department of Biostatistics and Data Science, Wake Forest School of Medicine, Medical Center Boulevard, Winston-Salem, NC 27157, USA
* Corresponding author.
E-mail address: scarmich@wakehealth.edu
Twitter: @scarmic8 (S.P.C.); @dm_kline (D.M.K.)

Surg Clin N Am 103 (2023) 233–245
https://doi.org/10.1016/j.suc.2022.11.001
0039-6109/23/© 2022 Elsevier Inc. All rights reserved.

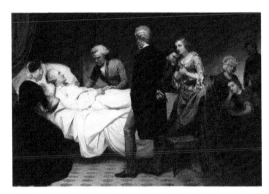

Fig. 1. Junius Brutus Stearns, American, 1810–1885. *Washington on his Deathbed,* 1851 Oil on canvas, 37 1/4 x 54 1/8 inches (94.62 x 137.48 cm) Dayton Art Institute, Dayton, Ohio. Gift of Mr. Robert Badenhop, 1954.16.

65. His property was extensive, and Washington rode on horseback approximately 6 hours each day to oversee his plantation's projects. On December 12, 1799, weather conditions turned poor with rain, snow, and sleet. In spite of this, Washington continued with his daily routine, subsequently experiencing chest congestion on the evening of the following day. He awoke the morning of December 14th with a sore throat and shortness of breath.[1] In the course of his ensuing illness which historians now believe to have been severe epiglottitis, Washington underwent multiple phlebotomies, toxic ingestions, herbal treatments, and cathartics in an effort to save his life.[2] Physicians, Drs James Craik, Gustavus Richard Brown, and Elisha Cullen Dick, were well-trained practitioners of their day and believed these modalities to represent best practices in the treatment of the former President. Nonetheless, their efforts were unsuccessful, and the first president of the United States succumbed to his illness at 10:20 PM on December 14, 1799.

The challenges at Washington's bedside transcend space and time. The same fundamental challenges faced by his treatment team are in play each day in thousands of hospital rooms across the world. His physicians undoubtedly had the same conversations: which intervention will have the best chance of success? What are the risks and benefits of each? When should we change our approach in the absence of a response? What would have happened if we made a different decision? Unfortunately, in any given decision tree, turning back the hands of time and introducing the same set of circumstances with the use of a different treatment (ie, the perfect counterfactual) is merely a thought experiment. Often, a combination of associations and extrapolated experiences is substituted for causality, the gold standard for decision-making evidence. The conclusion of a causal relationship is a rare indulgence, one that is classically exemplified in the public health literature with story of Dr John Snow and the pump handle.

Dr John Snow, considered the "Father of Epidemiology" for his investigations into the causes of cholera outbreaks and prevention of their recurrence, was an anesthesiologist in London, UK, during the mid-nineteenth century. He examined the patterns of infection during the cholera epidemic of 1854. The result was a detailed spot map of London's Golden Square area (**Fig. 2**). Believing cholera to be a water-borne illness, Snow made careful note of the local water pump stations on his map. Appreciating a density of disease around Pump A (ie, the Broad Street pump), he concluded that the disease must be arising from that location. Curiously, he also observed that no

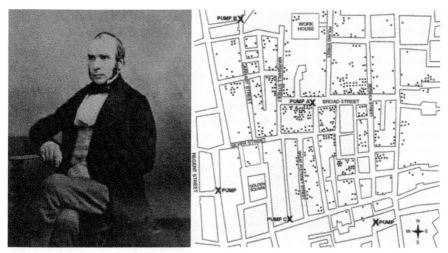

Fig. 2. Dr. John Snow (left). (Right) Map of the book "On the Mode of Communication of Cholera" by John Snow, originally published in 1854.

cases of cholera were identified among workers at a brewery two blocks east of Pump A. Dr Snow subsequently discovered that the workers used a well on the premises as their source of water rather than pump water. Given that the Broad Street pump was the common water source for the residents of Golden Square, Snow presented his findings to municipal officials and the pump handle was removed, concluding the outbreak.[3]

Although John Snow created a foundation for modern epidemiologic measurement, scientific investigation of clinical phenomenon rarely yields the luxury of "removing the pump handle" and the effort to determine causal relationships is typically more challenging. Instead, correlative relationships, where the intersection between a possible cause and effect is nebulous, are far more common, and investigators are left to postulate about which factors may be causal to the outcome. In this vein, Sir Bradford Hill (**Fig. 3**), an English economist, epidemiologist, and statistician, credited with pioneering the design of the modern randomized clinical trial, introduced his Causal Criteria in 1965.[4,5] These essential elements of determining a "cause" include strength of the association, consistency of the observed association, specificity (between cause and effect), temporality (cause precedes effect), biological gradient, plausibility, coherence (consistency with "generally known facts"), experiment, and analogy. Dr Hill comments:

"None of my nine viewpoints can bring indisputable evidence for or against the cause-and-effect hypothesis and none can be required as a sine qua non. What they can do, with greater or less strength, is to help us make up our minds on the fundamental question—is there any other way of explaining this set of facts before us, is there any other answer equally, or more, likely than cause and effect."[4]

Building on the work of Hill, Dr Kenneth Rothman (see **Fig. 3**), a professor of epidemiology at Boston University, introduced the Causal Pie Model in 1976. He defines *cause* as: "…an act or event or a state of nature which initiates or permits, alone or in conjunction with other causes, a sequence of events resulting in an effect."[6] From this approach, he discerns three different types of cause (**Fig. 4**). A *sufficient cause* is a set of conditions, without any one of which the disease would not have

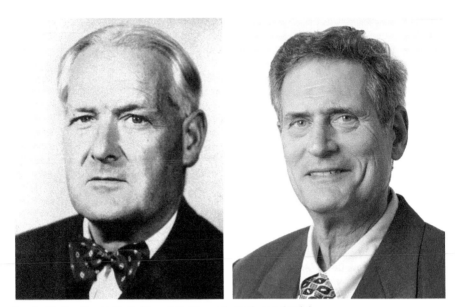

Fig. 3. Sir Bradford Hill (*left*) and Dr Kenneth Rothman (*right*).

occurred (ie, the whole pie). A *component* cause is any one of the set of conditions which are necessary for the completion of a sufficient cause (ie, a piece of the pie). A *necessary* cause is a component cause that is a member of every sufficient cause.

Taking these definitions together, several conclusions can be drawn from this model. First, the satisfaction of a sufficient cause makes the disease inevitable. Although this obviates the ability to prevent disease, the timeline for disease manifestation (ie, malignancy) may be prolonged, allowing for treatment to cure. Second, the component causes to create a sufficient cause may occur far apart in time, facilitating opportunities for preventative intervention. Last, blocking the action of any component cause prevents the completion of the sufficient cause, antagonizing the disease by that pathway.

Ultimately, the degree to which causal assertions of a given investigation is incorporated into surgical practice depends on the relationship between three factors: study design, data interpretation, and quality of care in surgery. This relationship may be expressed in the form of two questions:

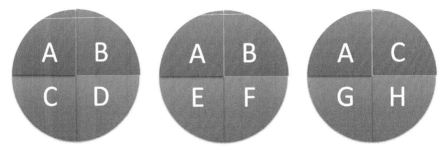

Fig. 4. Example of the Causal Pie Model. Sufficient cause: A+B+C+D; Component cause: A–D; Necessary cause: A.

1. Are the conclusions from a given investigation appropriately interpreted based on the study design?
2. Are the conclusions likely to yield improvements in quality of care in surgery?

If a study or trial is poorly designed, then its conclusions are uninterpretable. If the conclusions are unlikely to improve the quality of care, then they will not be incorporated into practice models for surgical decision-making. In turn, the levels (or categories) of evidence represent the degrees to which these questions are answered with decreasing amounts of bias and uncertainty. The following discussion will provide a framework of understanding for each of these three interrelated factors.

DISCUSSION
Quality of Care in Surgery

As Washington lay critically ill, the treatment practices of his physician team were being interrogated in Philadelphia. Benjamin Rush, a charismatic physician, statesman, and signer of the Declaration of Independence, was an ardent supporter of phlebotomy as a panacea for disease.[2] Craik, Brown, and Dick were all familiar with Rush. Craik and Rush served together in the Revolutionary War, Brown was his medical classmate in Edinburgh, and Dick was his trainee in Philadelphia.[7] For the past 2 years, Rush had been ensnared in a legal battle with William Cobbett, a journalist who alleged that Rush's enthusiastic blood-letting practice during the 1797 yellow fever epidemic in Philadelphia was tantamount to murder.[7] Although Cobbett was found guilty of libel (on the day of Washington's death), Rush never recovered his medical reputation and subsequently closed his practice. Fearing for their own reputations, Craik and Dick issued a statement to the nation following Washington's death, describing his illness and their treatment course. The article was negatively received with friends and members of the medical community suggesting that Washington was murdered.[2] Although phlebotomy was considered an accepted, yet heroic, therapy of the day, its treatment failure in this high-profile case called its utility into question.

Clinical research is fundamentally driven by outcomes. The Donabedian model, first proposed in the 1960s, provided a dynamic and generalizable assessment tool for the quality of health care via evaluation of structure, process, and outcomes.[8] Structure is the environment where care is being delivered and entails institutional, workforce and supply factors. Process is the coordination of care delivery, and outcomes are the effects of care delivered to the patient. Necessarily, outcomes are impacted by both structure and process. Allowing for selective evaluation in these separate elements, this model has been successfully applied to the care improvement of multiple different pathologies, including lung cancer, prostate cancer, congenital heart defects, and morbid obesity.[9]

The field of surgery began to systematically explore outcomes toward quality improvement in the 1990s and early 2000s by applying the Donabedian model to create both the National Surgical Quality Improvement Program (NSQIP) in the United States and the Physiological and Operative Severity Score for the Enumeration of Mortality and Morbidity in Europe.[10–13] NSQIP was originally birthed as the National Veterans Affairs Surgical Risk Study (NVASRS) and was developed in response to public criticism of the Department of Veterans Affairs (VA) for high operative mortality rates at the 133 VA hospitals in the 1980s.[14] Congress passed Public Law 99 to 166, mandating annual VA reporting of surgical outcomes on a comorbidity risk-adjusted basis for comparison to domestic averages. NVASRS collected preoperative, intraoperative, and 30-day postoperative outcome variables at 44 VA medical centers on more than 117,000 operations across nine surgical specialties from October 1991 to

December 1993.[14,15] The data correlated to the quality of structures and processes at the various centers and allowed the VA to improve postoperative mortality by 47% and morbidity by 43% across its system from 1991 to 2006.[15] NSQIP, established as an ongoing VA quality initiative following NVASRS, was subsequently piloted at several university institutions in 1999. The experiences of these non-VA centers validated the predictive and risk-adjusted models created by the VA in the heterogeneous patient population of the private sector.[15] Presently, the American College of Surgeons, as the managing body of NSQIP within the private sector, has enrolled more than 700 hospitals across the United States and over 100 hospitals internationally to its program, now the largest clinical general surgery registry in the world.[15]

Although national initiatives, such as NSQIP, have unquestionably improved the quality and standardization of surgical care, variations in surgical outcomes persist. Much to the chagrin of surgeons, patients, hospitals, insurance companies, and national agencies alike, there is no perfect metric for quality.[16] Importantly, in revisiting the Donabedian model, none of the three variables (ie, structure, process, or outcome) can be appropriately applied to evaluation of every procedure type. As demonstrated in **Fig. 5** from Ibrahim and Dimick, the quality metric used to asses a given operation is based on both the volume and risk associated with that procedure.[16]

Whereas high-risk/high-volume operations may be appropriately evaluated by their outcomes, low-risk/high-volume procedures (ie, laparoscopic cholecystectomy) would be unlikely to yield discriminatory outcomes between facilities.[17] The quality of these operations is likely best compared with process. Alternatively, procedures that are high-risk/low-volume may generate inadequate numbers at a given center

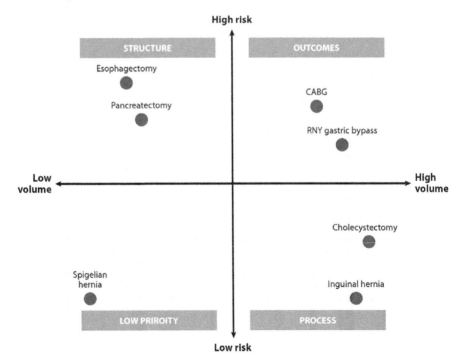

Fig. 5. Qualification of exemplary procedure types in correspondence with volume and risk. CABG, Coronary artery bypass graft; RNY, Roux-en-Y. (Reprinted with permission from Ibrahim AM, Dimick JB. What Metrics Accurately Reflect Surgical Quality? Annu Rev Med. 2018;69:481-491.)

to accurately compare outcomes. Therefore, quality may be measured in the variable of structure (ie, volume of operations), which is supported by prior work.[18,19]

Because of the limitations described in traditional quality assessments, exploration of new metrics is an imperative. As the surgical field is fundamentally interventional, there is inherently human variable of quality in performance. Based on intraoperative video monitoring, differences in technical skills may influence outcomes.[20] Comparison based on this modality could yield standardization in technique and training, a variable yet to be included within the graduate surgical education frameworks of the United States.[21,22] Furthermore, patient-reported outcomes, or the quality-of-life assessments following operation, could inform traditional outcome measurements. Although there is popular agreement that these should be included, the processes for their collection and evaluation remain unstandardized.[16]

The evolution of the Donabedian concept has provided surgical researchers a framework by which quality of care may be evaluated. However, a proper study design remains crucial for durable progress to be made in these categories. Data that are collected in response to flawed hypotheses, gathered inappropriately, and applied incorrectly frustrate improvements in surgical care. Thus, it is on surgeons to evaluate the literature for appropriate conclusions based on the study design before updating practice models for surgical decision-making.

Study Design and Levels of Evidence

Clinical research in surgery is generated primarily from analytical study designs, though case reports are frequently written on interesting or uncommon topics to generate awareness. Interpretation of outcomes from a case report is extremely limited, not generalizable and should frame what is *possible* rather than what is *probable*. Beyond anecdotal reports, the two general categories of medical research include experimental and observational designs. Observational designs are commonly referred to as "studies," whereas experimental designs are termed "trials," as they include some form of assigned intervention. In general, the quality of evidence from the hierarchy in **Fig. 6** is inversely proportional to the level of potential bias within a given design. Generally defined, bias is "any systematic error in the design, conduct, or analysis of a study that results in a mistaken estimate" or "any tendency which prevents unprejudiced consideration of a question."[23,24] Bias may occur at all phases of a trial or study, influencing study design, data collection, analysis, and interpretation.

Epidemiologic observational studies can be divided into three categories: cohort studies, case-control studies, and cross-sectional studies. Observational studies may be prospective or retrospective and are ideal in circumstances where a given intervention may be unethical to assign to participants (ie, cigarettes, alcohol). Rather than introducing an exposure, participants in prospective cohort studies are chosen based on their current exposure status and followed over a period to assess incidence of a variety of outcomes. The primary rationale for this type of study is to learn about the health effects of an exposure. The relationship between the exposure and the disease state is expressed in terms of relative risk (or risk ratio). Especially, the incidence of a given outcome is compared as a ratio of rates between the exposed and unexposed (control) groups. The major value of cohort studies is in their evaluation of multiple outcomes, particularly for rare exposures. Their limitation is the inability to study multiple exposures, as a single exposure is typically the basis for study inclusion. Prospective cohort studies are also a poor choice for diseases that take a long time to manifest or are very rare, as few outcomes may be observed during the study period. An alternative design, commonly used in surgical research, is the retrospective cohort study where the exposure and outcome have already been

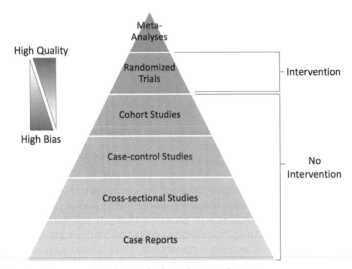

Fig. 6. Clinical evidence quality hierarchy based on study type.

observed. This allows for the choice of an exposure without a delay in measuring outcomes, which can reduce the burden of running a prospective study. However, as data for these studies are largely gleaned from electronic medical records and administrative databases, they are typically not collecting data for research and are prone to multiple biases related to selection, recall, misclassification, and missing data. While having great potential to advance research, electronic medical records and other administrative databases come with challenges that require their own consideration when designing studies.[25,26] One useful framework for conceptualizing the design of observational studies is to emulate a target trial (ie, the trial that would be run in an ideal world).[27]

Case-control studies are always retrospective and begin with the selection of a single outcome (ie, disease) rather than a single exposure. Here, the key research question is, "Given your outcome status, did you previously have the exposure of interest?" Importantly, controls must have the opportunity to have developed the disease of interest. For instance, a group of men would not be an appropriate control for uterine cancer incidence in a sample of women. The results of a relationship between disease and exposure in case-control studies are expressed as an odds ratio, as risk between exposure and outcome cannot be directly established. As case-control studies sample based on the outcome of interest, they are good tools for rare diseases and diseases with long latencies, taking into account multiple exposures. A weakness of case-control studies is their inability to look at multiple outcomes, inability to directly measure risk based on exposure, and susceptibility to bias from choice of controls. Matching of cases and controls is common in case-control studies to increase statistical efficiency, but such choices should be carefully thought through and evaluated to avoid unintended consequences.[28]

Cross-sectional studies look at a population sample during a single time point, like a "snapshot" in time. Alternatively, they may be followed up with repeated measures over multiple time points (repeated cross-sectional or panel study). The main purpose of this design type is to answer questions about the prevalence (ie, how many cases) or incidence (ie, how many new cases in a repeated measure design) of a given disease within the population of interest. The strengths of cross-sectional studies are in their ability to describe multiple variables within a population.[29] They frequently contain large sample sizes and serve as preliminary data for planning of future investigation. As they ascertain exposure and outcome at the same time, the ability of cross-sectional studies to suggest causality is limited. A flow chart to assist with study definition is listed in **Fig. 7**.[30]

Methods of Interpretation

If the data needed to assist surgeons with making the best quality of care decisions for patients come from a variety of study designs, how do we decide which data to adopt and which to reject? One way is with a directed acyclic graph (DAG).[31] A DAG provides a visual representation of the assumed model and relationships between variables of interest (**Fig. 8**). Through the effective use of DAGs, one can identify potential sources of bias (ie, confounders) during the study design phase and select appropriate analyses to mitigate such bias. Creating a DAG can also be a helpful exercise when interpreting the published literature, allowing for critical evaluation of hypotheses, achievement of stated outcomes and clinical relevance.

After settling on a causal model and a target quantity (ie, estimand) of interest, one must consider the balance between accuracy (bias) and precision (variance). As shown in **Fig. 9**, the ideal case is of high accuracy and high precision where estimates are tightly centered on the target. In practice, accuracy of an estimator is often determined by the design and analytical strategy, whereas precision is largely determined by sample size. Owing to the link between precision and sample size, it is important to be aware of the big data paradox, which notes that, despite increasing precision, small biases are often compounded with increasing sample sizes.[32,33] In surgery, this paradox could arise from the use of large claims or electronic health record databases

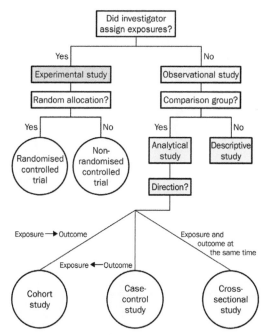

Fig. 7. Flow chart for definition of clinical research designs. (Reprinted with permission from Elsevier. The Lancet, Jan 2002, 359 (9300), 57–61.)

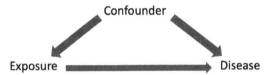

Fig. 8. Directed acyclic graph format demonstrating the relationship between exposure and disease. A confounder is a variable not on the causal pathway but associated with both the exposure and disease.

that are subject to inherent structural biases. In other words, data quality is often more important than data quantity for generating high-quality evidence.

Most importantly, the interpretation of study results is based on notions of statistical and clinical significance. Statistical significance is typically determined by the result of a null hypothesis test. Hypothesis testing assumes a null hypothesis in the causal model and typically, no effect of treatment. A P value is calculated to determine the probability that one would observe data as extreme or more extreme than what was actually observed, assuming the null hypothesis model is true. If the P value is small enough, the null hypothesis is rejected because it is unlikely that the data would have been observed if the null hypothesis was actually true. Confidence intervals provide another way of illustrating uncertainty around a parameter estimate and are linked to hypothesis tests. Confidence intervals show the set of parameters that would be compatible with the data observed.[34] For example, a confidence interval of (−1, 2) would be compatible with a null hypothesis, inclusive of 0, but also null hypotheses of all effects in the interval from −1 to 2.

It is critical to examine whether an estimated statistical effect is relevant to clinical practice. Although one could identify increasingly small statistically significant effects in large sample sizes, those differences only remain clinically meaningful to a point. It is up to the surgeon to determine the minimal clinically important difference (MCID) for

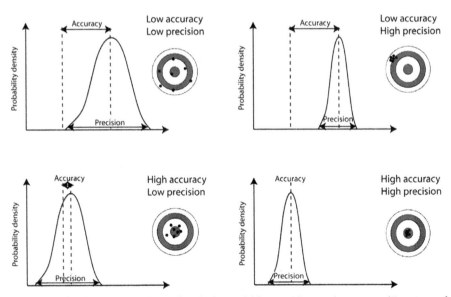

Fig. 9. Graphical representations of variations within precision and accuracy. (*Courtesy of* Dr. Bethan Davis, AntarcticGlaciers.org.)

their estimand. The determination of the MCID should be planned before data collection for an appropriate power calculation and to prevent unnecessary data collection.

Several important fallacies can arise while interpreting results. The vast majority can be prevented by preplanning, pre-specification, and preregistration of the design, outcomes, and analysis plan. The determination of statistical power, a function of variability and sample size, is a key part of this preparation to ensure appropriate decision-making about the primary endpoints based on the study design characteristics. Power calculations are not useful after an analysis (post hoc power) or to argue for the truth of the null hypothesis.[35] It should be noted that absence of evidence against the null hypothesis is not evidence of absence of an effect. Other fallacies related to multiple testing, p-hacking, and selective presentation of results can also be mitigated through rigorous planning and pre-specification.[36]

SUMMARY

The death of George Washington illustrates the struggle that physicians and surgeons face on a regular basis—the persistent and inherent duality of critically appraising the literature and applying it to the patient at the bedside. Washington's physicians had no intention of expediting his demise. It was their causal model and evidence structure that was incorrect. Unfortunately, the challenge of the counterfactual persists through time—we cannot go back and try a different treatment under the same set of circumstances. Bias exists everywhere and there is no such thing as a "bias-free" study design that perfectly applies to every clinical scenario. It is upon us to be able to interpret the contemporary data and evolve our practices with the best evidence we have. In this way, the final hours of Washington's life serve as both the narrative of our history in medicine and the plow to which we must set our hands.

CLINICS CARE POINTS

- The degree to which causal assertions are incorporated into surgical practice depends on the relationship between study design, data interpretation and quality of care in surgery.
- Data that are collected in response to flawed hypotheses, gathered inappropriately, and applied incorrectly frustrate improvements in surgical care.
- Bias is a tendency which prevents unprejudiced consideration of a question and may occur at all phases of a trial or study, influencing design, data collection, analysis, and interpretation.
- Directed acyclic graphs provide a visual representation of the assumed model and relationships between variables of interest.
- The accuracy of an estimator is often determined by the study design and analytical strategy, whereas precision is largely determined by sample size.
- It is critical to examine whether an estimated statistical effect is relevant to clinical practice with the determination of the minimal clinically important difference (MCID) prior to data collection.

ACKNOWLEDGMENTS

The authors wish to appreciate the thoughtful review of this article from Drs Lucas P. Neff, Department of Pediatric Surgery, Wake Forest School of Medicine and Michael Chang, Chief Medical Officer and Associate Vice President for Medical Affairs, University of Southern Alabama.

DISCLOSURE

The project described was supported by the National Center for Advancing Translational Sciences, National Institutes of Health, through Grant KL2TR001421. The content is solely the responsibility of the authors and does not necessarily represent the official views of the NIH.

REFERENCES

1. Kort A. George Washington's Final Years - And Sudden, Agonizing Death. History. 2020. Available at: https://www.history.com/news/george-washington-final-years-death-mount-vernon. Accessed March 22, 2022.
2. Morens DM. Death of a President. N Engl J Med 2008;341(24):1845–50.
3. Lesson 1: Introduction to Epidemiology. CDC. 2012. Available at: https://www.cdc.gov/csels/dsepd/ss1978/Lesson1/Section2.html#_ref5. Accessed March 22, 2022.
4. Hill AB. The environment and disease: association or causation? Proc R Soc Med 1965;58(5):295–300.
5. Doll R. Sir Austin Bradford Hill and the progress of medical science. BMJ Br Med J 1992;305(6868):1521.
6. Rothman KJ. Causes. Am J Epidemiol 1976;104(6):587–92.
7. North RL. Benjamin Rush, MD: assassin or beloved healer? Proc (Bayl Univ Med Cent) 2000;13(1):45.
8. Donabedian A. Evaluating the quality of medical care. Milbank Q 2005;83(4): 691–729.
9. Santry HP, Strassels SA, Ingraham AM, et al. Identifying the fundamental structures and processes of care contributing to emergency general surgery quality using a mixed-methods Donabedian approach. BMC Med Res Methodol 2020; 20(1):1–19.
10. Peskin GW. Quality care in surgery. Arch Surg 2002;137(1):13–4.
11. Marti MC, Roche B. Quality control in outpatient surgery: what data are useful? Ambul Surg 1998;6(1):21–3.
12. Copeland GP, Jones D, Walters M. POSSUM: a scoring system for surgical audit. Br J Surg 1991;78(3):355–60.
13. Khuri SF, Daley J, Henderson W, et al. Risk adjustment of the postoperative mortality rate for the comparative assessment of the quality of surgical care: results of the National Veterans Affairs Surgical Risk Study. J Am Coll Surg 1997;185(4): 315–27.
14. Khuri SF, Daley J, Henderson WG. The comparative assessment and improvement of quality of surgical care in the department of veterans affairs. Arch Surg 2002;137(1):20–7.
15. History of ACS NSQIP. American College of Surgeons. 2022. Available at: https://www.facs.org/quality-programs/acs-nsqip/about/history. Accessed March 25, 2022.
16. Ibrahim AM, Dimick JB. What metrics accurately reflect surgical quality? Annu Rev Med 2018;69:481–91.
17. Ibrahim AM, Hughes TG, Thumma JR, et al. Association of hospital critical access status with surgical outcomes and expenditures among medicare beneficiaries. JAMA 2016;315(19):2095–103.
18. Birkmeyer JD, Stukel TA, Siewers AE, et al. Surgeon volume and operative mortality in the United States. N Engl J Med 2003;349(22):2117–27.

19. Birkmeyer JD, Siewers AE, Finlayson EVA, et al. Hospital volume and surgical mortality in the United States. N Engl J Med 2002;346(15):1128–37.
20. Birkmeyer JD, Finks JF, O'Reilly A, et al. Surgical skill and complication rates after bariatric surgery. N Engl J Med 2013;369(15):1434–42.
21. Habuchi T, Terachi T, Mimata H, et al. Evaluation of 2,590 urological laparoscopic surgeries undertaken by urological surgeons accredited by an endoscopic surgical skill qualification system in urological laparoscopy in Japan. Surg Endosc 2012;26(6):1656–63.
22. Tanigawa N, Lee SW, Kimura T, et al. The endoscopic surgical skill qualification system for gastric surgery in Japan. Asian J Endosc Surg 2011;4(3):112–5.
23. Pannucci CJ, Wilkins EG. Identifying and avoiding bias in research. Plast Reconstr Surg 2010;126(2):619.
24. Schlesselman JJ, Stolley PD. Case-control studies : design, conduct, analysis. New York: Oxford University Press; 1982.
25. Shortreed SM, Cook AJ, Coley RY, et al. Challenges and opportunities for using big health care data to advance medical science and public health. Am J Epidemiol 2019;188(5):851–61.
26. Casey JA, Schwartz BS, Stewart WF, et al. Using electronic health records for population health research: a review of methods and applications. Annu Rev Public Health 2016;37:61–81.
27. Hernán MA, Robins JM. Using big data to emulate a target trial when a randomized trial is not available. Am J Epidemiol 2016;183(8):758–64.
28. Mansournia MA, Jewell NP, Greenland S, et al. Case-control matching: effects, misconceptions, and recommendations. Eur J Epidemiol 2018;33(1):5–14.
29. Wang X, Cheng Z. Cross-sectional studies: strengths, weaknesses, and recommendations. Chest 2020;158(1):S65–71.
30. Grimes DA, Schulz KF. An overview of clinical research: the lay of the land. Lancet (London, England) 2002;359(9300):57–61.
31. Lipsky AM, Greenland S. Causal directed acyclic graphs. JAMA 2022;327(11):1083–4.
32. Meng XL. Statistical paradises and paradoxes in big data (I): law of large populations, big data paradox, and the 2016 US presidential election. Ann Appl Stat 2018;12(2):685–726.
33. Bradley VC, Kuriwaki S, Isakov M, et al. Unrepresentative big surveys significantly overestimated US vaccine uptake. Nature 2021;600(7890):695–700.
34. Greenland S, Senn SJ, Rothman KJ, et al. Statistical tests, P values, confidence intervals, and power: a guide to misinterpretations. Eur J Epidemiol 2016;31(4):337.
35. Hoenig JM, Heisey DM. The abuse of power. Am Stat 2012;55(1):19–24.
36. Nuzzo R. How scientists fool themselves - and how they can stop. Nature 2015;526(7572):182–5.

Clinical Informatics and the Electronic Medical Record

Mustafa Abid, MD, Andrew B. Schneider, MD, MSc*

KEYWORDS

- Electronic medical record • Informatics • Surgeons

KEY POINTS

- Although electronic medical record (EMR) use can lead to increased provider documentation burden, adjuncts including scribes, voice recognition software, and smart templating can help to offset.
- Data gathered through the EMR can enable better clinical deterioration tools, operating room scheduling tools, and decision support systems.
- Informatics is still in its infancy within surgery and has the potential to revolutionize the field.

INTRODUCTION

The electronic medical record (EMR) is ubiquitous to clinical care across specialties, hospitals, and health care systems in the United States and increasingly globally. Today's surgeon relies on the EMR to access patient records, place orders, schedule operations, track patient laboratory values and vital signs, and communicate with both patients and staff.

Integral to the utilization of the EMR to affect patient outcomes, clinical informatics represents a broad and growing field involving data utilization and management often in the service of various research efforts, now bolstered by the rapid growth in advanced machine learning and artificial intelligence.

Both the EMR and clinical informatics are two topics not often conflated with the practice of surgery. Although these elements of surgery may be viewed through the paradigm of "research" or as siloed away from clinical surgical practice, they in fact shape surgical practice and a working knowledge of how to use these tools to advance patient care represents a valuable and integral addition to every surgeon's toolkit.

Department of Surgery, University of North Carolina, 101 Manning Drive, Chapel Hill, NC 27514, USA
* Corresponding author.
E-mail address: andrew_schneider@med.unc.edu

Surg Clin N Am 103 (2023) 247–258
https://doi.org/10.1016/j.suc.2022.11.005

HISTORY OF THE ELECTRONIC MEDICAL RECORD

EMRs are so ingrained in medical practice today that it is difficult to fathom a time before their existence. Before their widespread usage, paper charting dominated the inpatient and ambulatory settings. Endless storage rooms of unorganized illegible records were common. Requests to ascertain old imaging results or transfers of entire medical records to other facilities had massive backlogs and could take weeks to months before being fulfilled.

In the later part of the twentieth-century computer server cost and footprint started to rapidly decrease. The Institute of Medicine in 1991 recognized the potential impact of electronic record keeping and issued a report: "Computer-based Patient Records: An Essential Technology for Health Care." This landmark paper provided an assessment of current paper-based medical record systems and provided a framework to convert to an electronic medium. In 2009, the US Congress passed the Health Information Technology for Economic and Clinical Health Act, which monetarily incentivized physicians and hospitals to use EMRs and penalized those who resisted. With the implementation of electronic records tied to reimbursement, multiple health care technology start-ups sprouted overnight. The use of the EMR increased from 12.2% of US hospitals in 2009 to 75.5% in 2014 to over 95% in 2017.[1,2]

Today, only a handful of the initial hundreds of medical record companies continue to exist. Most non-government-based inpatient hospitals have a limited choice of software packages to use as the market share is dominated by this small subset of companies.

REVIEW OF CLINICAL INFORMATICS AND ELECTRONIC MEDICAL RECORD TERMINOLOGY

Data science: A field focused on how to create knowledge from data.[3]

Electronic medical record: An electronic patient medical chart—this is modifiable and inclusive of medical, demographic, and administrative data.[4]

Real-world evidence: Data regarding patient's health or health services data derived from the EMR, insurance and billing data, patient generated data, mobile devices, and so forth.[5]

Clinical Informatics

The American Medical Informatics Association defines clinical informatics as "the application of informatics and information technology to deliver health care services," whereas the UK Faculty of Clinical Informatics defines a clinical informatician as, "[Someone who] uses their clinical knowledge and experience of informatics concepts, methods, and tools to promote patient and population care that is person-centered, ethical, safe, effective, efficient, timely, and equitable."[6]

Applied clinical informatics includes the analysis, design, implementation, and evaluation of information systems with the goal of improving both individual and population-level health outcomes.[7]

Surgical Data Science

A field whose objective is to improve surgical health care by learning how to accurately and descriptively capture data on interventions and patient health status intraoperative and perioperative and applying these lessons to improve decision-making processes perioperatively and intraoperatively.[3,8]

Surgical quality improvement has often used case-based reviews including Morbidity and Mortality conference.[8] Registry studies and other large databases have been increasingly used to evaluate surgical quality through pooled outcomes measures and to develop real-time tools such as risk calculators.[8] However, the rate of surgical complications remains high even with these efforts.[3] As clinical informatics has grown and the volume of potential data actively generated during surgical procedures has increased, new applications for clinical informatics have emerged.

This subfield of clinical informatics has been coined "Surgical Data Science." This term encompasses not only the patient and their related data but also the clinical team caring for the patient, devices used in their care, dynamic monitoring of vitals as well as laboratory values and procedural data, and finally "domain knowledge" including system guidelines and workflows and lessons learned from prior interventions.[3] These categories represent significant, previously unused or underused sources of data. Capturing and analyzing these data provide a much larger pool of evidence for surgeons to draw on when they want to study the factors contributing to their operative outcomes, both perioperatively and intraoperatively.

REVIEW OF MACHINE LEARNING

Increasingly ubiquitous in discussions about data collection, cleaning, analysis, and application, the term "Machine Learning" bears at least brief mention here. Machine learning differs from traditional computer programs because the latter is "rules based," whereas the former is based in experiential learning.[9] The goal is to let the computer "learn" to define and classify the data without providing predefined rules.[9] The larger the data set, the more accurate the machine learning algorithm.[9] The underlying theorems, methodology, and implementation are beyond the scope of this article, but it is important that the reader understands the terminology to decipher the origins of the tool in the EMR. Please see the accompanying article Shruthi Srinivas and Andrew Young's article, "Machine Learning and Artificial Intelligence in Surgical Research," in this issue for a more comprehensive overview of the topic.

APPLYING THE ELECTRONIC MEDICAL RECORD TO CHALLENGES IN SURGERY
Predicting Clinical Deterioration

Surgical risk calculators such as the American College of Surgeons National Surgical Quality Improvement Program and the American Society of Anesthesiologists classification system provide important perioperative risk assessment using static preoperative variables. These models were developed based on historical pooled data and cannot account for dynamic postoperative changes once patients reach the surgical floors, limiting their ability to pinpoint the time points at which the risk of clinical deterioration are greatest. More recently, risk prediction models for nonsurgical patients have been developed using EHR data including trends in vitals, laboratory values, and clinical assessment of the patient to accurately predict clinical deterioration events.[10] The breadth and granularity of data available in the EHR enabled the development of more accurate risk prediction tools, including the Modified Early Warning Score, National Early Warning Score, and electronic Cardiac Arrest Risk Triage (eCART) score.[11] These tools can then be tested retrospectively against tens of thousands of patients, again using the large volume of data points and variables in the EHR to validate their use. One of these tools, eCART, uses greater than 30 dynamic variables to predict clinical deterioration.[11] Every time there is a new result for a variable in the model (new blood pressure, new creatinine, and so forth); the model generates a new deterioration risk score enabling physicians to avert catastrophic patient decompensation with early interventions in real time.

Estimating Operating Room Case Time

The operating room, and more specifically how it is used, drives both hospital revenue and cost. Efficient scheduling allows for care to be provided to greater numbers of patients, inefficiencies in scheduling often leave ORs underused or misused, driving both delays of surgical care and hospital cost.[12] Although using the EMR for electronic OR scheduling has been shown to shorten patient length of stay, the current methods for developing these time estimates have limitations and opportunities for improvement.[13] Previous strategies, including surgeons self-submitting case time estimates or averaging case times in the EMR, have both been shown to be inaccurate.[12] These self-estimations of OR utilization are prone to significant bias, relying on nonspecific data including CPT codes rather than on patient or case-specific factors. Surgeon and service-specific models have been developed using a data set of greater than 40,000 cases, focusing on patient-specific data points that influenced the difference in operative time for the same posted case, with improved accuracy over surgeon or previous EMR-based scheduler produced operative time predictions.[12] Various other machine-learning-based scheduling programs have reduced errors in time estimates by between 15% and 40%.[14,15] Other efforts have targeted not only prediction of surgery duration but also of postoperative anesthesia time.[16] Further optimization of scheduling prediction may include dynamic predictions of case duration based on intraoperative data, not just relying on previous surgeon time averages.[3] The result of these efforts, rooted in the large volumes of data collected through the EMR but enhanced by current methods of data analytics including machine learning, will be to optimize OR schedules to ensure more cases are completed in the available OR time, with less overruns and overtime staffing needs.

Electronic Medical Record/Informatics and Reimbursement

Any discussion focused on the EMR and clinical informatics must cover the basic finances that have driven and currently drive EMR implementation and adoption, modification, and standards of use. As discussed earlier, the major turning point in EMR utilization in the United States came in 2009 as the result of legislative mandates for EMR adoption nationally. However, the economics of the EMR have always featured prominently in discussions regarding its adoption and use. Financial incentives were offered by the federal government at that time to enable EMR adoption and to address concerns about short-term economic downsides to a transition from paper to electronic records.[17] The implementation of the EMR in large and small practices across the United States, while now ubiquitous, faced and continues to face criticism that the required data input actually slows down practices and reduces productivity, and by extension impacts revenue. Much of the early research focused on determining the impact of the EMR on clinical productivity produced mixed results.[17,18] Interestingly, many of the studies conducted before 2009 demonstrated some financial benefit to EMR implementation.[17] This may suggest that when applied on a case-by-case basis at timing determined by health systems, EMR implementation did provide financial benefits over paper charting. It is difficult to definitively determine though, as the volume of EMR adoption remained low before 2009, limiting the data available for analysis.

These early studies found several specific contributors to cost reduction and revenue increases. The EMR helped to reduce redundant orders by over 20% in one study, whereas another demonstrated 12.7% overall cost reduction for each admission in the studied hospital.[17] Before implementation of EMR systems, there were few automated monitoring and determent systems to prevent repeat or redundant tests. Written orders could be submitted and implemented despite being a duplicate. EMR systems allow for automated soft and hard stops at the time of order entry, identifying for users duplicate orders and requesting users reconcile the duplicates or confirm that the duplicate order was intentional. Further, given the increased ease with which information is accessed, providers can quickly review years of medical records, filter searching them to find specific evaluations, laboratory and imaging results, allowing them to better determine the timing and utility of repeating tests.

Early studies of EMR cost effects also found that revenue could be increased by EMR implementation through more accurate and comprehensive capture of billing codes.[17] Previous work before EMR implementation had demonstrated up to 15% loss of billing revenue due to incomplete or improperly coded billing.[17] Other studies, demonstrated significant net revenue gains for systems with a positive, linear correlation to the amount a system invested in its information technology systems, including the EMR.[17] The numerous studies before wide scale implementation of the EMR, while presenting a multifaceted picture of the economic impacts of EMR utilization, seemed to provide ample evidence of a beneficial effect for health system finances. The evidence from the first several years following 2009 provided a more mixed picture. This, however, may not have been unanticipated, given that the legislation driving EMR implementation itself recognized that there may be short-term financial downsides to EMR adoption and provided financial incentives to attempt to offset this concern for health systems.

One more recent, single-center, multi-practice study demonstrated that although clinical productivity decreased with EMR implementation, practice-wide reimbursements increased, suggesting higher reimbursement per patient after EMR implementation.[18] More recent reviews of the literature have demonstrated a mixed picture. Although some reviewed studies demonstrated both increased provider productivity as well as increased revenue, others demonstrated the opposite, with significant decreases in physician productivity after implementation of the EMR.[19,20] Likewise, research has produced mixed results regarding increased or decreased charting workload following EMR implementation. Some work has found that specific types of billable encounters increased following EMR implementation, including ancillary procedures in one study and critical care billing in another.[18,20] Reviews at the system level have likewise produced mixed results. Some reviews have not found an association between EHR implementation and increased revenue at the hospital system level, although they demonstrated improvements in clinical scores tracking efficiency and patient quality.[21] Other studies have, however, demonstrated a positive association between EMR implementation and hospital financial performance.[22]

Some of this discordance in the data may be due to a lag effect between initial EMR implementation and the point at which providers achieve optimal EMR use. A similar delayed effect has been documented in other health technologies when they were likewise studied to determine financial benefit and also well documented in earlier EMR studies that found a lag of several years between EMR implementation and positive effects on efficiency and revenue.[22] Optimal use does not occur immediately after staff have completed EMR training, but requires time, personalization of EMR user interfaces, and recognition of initial shortcomings.

The time required for providers to learn and apply optimized documentation strategies further delays appreciable financial benefits from the EMR. As providers became more facile with the EMR, they became better able to apply billing codes to their encounters.[18,20] Further, as providers become more familiar with their EMR interface and how to customize it, they develop time-saving features including templates for documentation that capture all appropriate billing codes as well as preprepared order sets which expedite the input of patient orders. These small changes, though impactful in patient throughput and appropriate billing, require time and provider comfort with the EMR. It is not unreasonable to suspect that as the number of providers who have trained only with the EMR increases, this will drive further optimization of EMR systems and result in more easily demonstrated reimbursement benefits to EMR usage.

LIMITATIONS TO ELECTRONIC MEDICAL RECORD
Data Conformity and the Electronic Medical Record

The utilization of EMR data for Surgical Data Science and improving surgical outcomes continues to be limited by and despite the vast, heterogeneous data available in the EMR. The EMR contains enormous quantities of patient data from both static sources such as clinical assessments, patient surveys, and laboratories, but also hemodynamic monitoring and even intraoperative motion capture.[8] In surgical fields, majority of these data are not stored in a standardized, accessible format that would enable analysis.[3] Attempts to standardize data input or make that data more accessible must also balance the risk of increasing documentation burden on the already documentation-fatigued surgeon of the twenty-first century.[9] The approaches to improve standardization include more uniformly formatted data input and using AI to improve data extraction programs.

EMR interoperability poses another barrier to maximizing the available data for both patient care and research purposes. Interoperability challenges can manifest as inability to access outside imaging, transfer of clinical data from an integrated format in one EMR context to free text in another, and failure of transmission of electronic cancellation of medications to both pharmacies and other EMRs linked to the same patient.[23] Although beyond the scope of this article, several approaches to improve EHR interoperability demonstrate promise. Frameworks to support interoperability, including Fast Healthcare Interoperability Resources and Health Level 7, seek to create standards for EHR information exchange and increasingly also rely on blockchain-based technologies to facilitate secure interoperability of systems.[24,25] The goal of these efforts is to overcome some of the fragmentation in data sharing providers encountered in the current environment, which is characterized by multiple different EMRs across different health systems, which may differ even if these systems contract from the same EMR provider.

Bias and the Electronic Medical Record

Bias should be central to any discussions about the limitations of clinical informatics and the EMR. Dr Lesly Dossett provides a more comprehensive discussion of bias and cognitive dissonance in surgery in part ten of this collection. The pervasiveness of bias in the utilization of EMR data has been well-documented.[9,26–28] Bias in the EHR, data analytics, and machine learning is rooted in the biases present in the core data itself. Both unconscious bias and intentional bias affect how data are selected and curated for entry, how data analysis topics are chosen and how analytical models are constructed.[9] Data may be biased by patient selection, old practices in treatment or data recording, and disparities in how conditions are qualitatively or quantitatively described between different patients.[9] The EHR data are also biased by the dependence on medical billing coding for data input, selection of which data should or should not be recorded, patients lost to follow-up being excluded for analysis, and disparate access to systems with different EMRs.[1] Inputting biased data into a machine learning system would then increase the risk that those biases carry forward into the data analysis the machine learning program generates.[9]

To counter the many risks posed by bias in the EMR and related data analytics, models and programs developed from these large pools of data need to be validated in trials to confirm a lack of bias. Further, the providers using these systems will need the training to ensure they can recognize these biases and the risks they pose to accurate data analysis.[9] Compiling data from multiple EHRs across different health systems may help alleviate some of these risks for bias.

Security and the Electronic Medical Record

Although collecting large volumes of data presents opportunities for the advancement of research, it also creates vulnerability for data security. Recent reporting from the Department of Health and Human Services provides a stark reminder of the security threats facing patient information. In 2021, 578 health care organizations reported patient data breaches involving over 41 million patients;[29] 38 of these breaches each involved over 2 million patients.[29] In addition to the numerous risks, these data breaches pose to patient privacy and safety, and they also create a significant financial burden on systems, with average costs of a health care information breach reaching over $9 million each.[29] Recognizing the severity of these challenges means recognizing that effective data security requires a cohesive, interdisciplinary approach applied across all stakeholders in an EHR system.

It is important to involve institutional review boards (IRB) in data security when EHR data are used for research. The IRB will facilitate limited access to the data through certifications, audit logs, and data use agreements while also facilitating centrally located data repositories to facilitate improved data security.[30] All data that can be anonymized should, while data that cannot be de-identified must have its access carefully managed through data management plans created by the research team in consultation with the IRB.[30]

EMR security is made more complex by the rapidly growing volume of data to be secured, the need to share these data across entities, and the incorporation of cloud computing services into health data management.[31] The implementation of blockchain technologies, similar in concept to those used in the now popularized cryptocurrency space, offers one solution to improve EMR security while enabling large volumes of data to be shared across health care entities. Although beyond the scope of this article, blockchain's role in the future of EMR security is currently a topic of active research.[31,32] As efforts to improve EMR security grow in their complexity and gain more impetus from legislative requirements for protecting patient information, these efforts may hinder attempts to improve the interoperability of EMR systems both within and between health systems.[33] Stakeholders will have to grapple with balancing the evolving health information security needs posed by the EMR with competing needs to make its operation and interoperability less complex.

The Electronic Medical Record, Documentation Burden, and Burnout

Although many benefits of the EMR have been described, providers have experienced that the EMR and its documentation requirements, including admission and progress notes, discharge paperwork, and so forth, can be onerous. One group found that almost half of their hospital charges and over half of their work relative value units came from documentation, with that documentation accounting for over 1500 hours of labor in 1 year.[34] Other studies have estimated that almost half of provider time is now spent using the EHR or other administrative task work.[35] Many providers, both inside and outside of surgery, have found these documentation demands continuing into their post-work hours, and this is often pointed to as a contributing cause of burnout.[34–36]

The mixture of regulatory requirements and increased documentation needs within the EMR compared with previous paper charting methods have contributed to this significant increase in expected documentation. The workload that this documentation creates is compounded by gaps between perceived and actual EMR usability, a static approach to EMR design and implementation, and a paradigm that initially focused on individual provider usage of the EMR instead of on how the EMR integrated into the entire patient care pathway.[37] This has been reflected in poor "usability scores" that have not shown significant improvement with time, despite legislative efforts to compel improved EMR usability from vendors.[38] EMR usability challenges are influenced by pre-implementation testing during the product design period, training of users during the implementation period, and what elements of a vendor's EMR each health facility chooses to deploy.[38] The current literature indicates that increasing the availability of on-site EMR service staff in addition to increased IT support improves provider perceptions of the EMR and reduces symptoms of burnout.[39] Further, providers are not consistently included in EMR development, implementation, or improvement efforts.[39] Without significant provider input, EMR design may result in redundant workflows, the absence of clinically necessary tools, and processes that while perceived as streamlined in development are, in clinical implementation, bulky and even obstructive to the in vivo flow of clinical care.

Intentional, outcome-oriented structures to promote provider engagement in identifying and improving shortcomings in the EMR create critical stakeholder buy-in and enable more effective and durable solutions. Previously published experiences using an interdisciplinary team including providers to identify and implement changes in their EMR system not only resulted in numerous EMR improvements but also in self-reported physician proficiency with the EMR system.[40]

Providers have also noted that some regulatory requirements have increased documentation and data entry burden for EMR users. Owing to provider advocacy, changes at the federal level now seek to diminish documentation requirements. Recent changes through the Centers for Medicare and Medicaid services in implementing the "Patients over Paperwork" program seek to decrease some of the existing documentation requirements for Evaluation and Management services.[39]

One promising and well-studied solution to this challenge is the utilization of scribes or non-medically trained staff who assist with documentation. In a study undertaken by a trauma surgery group at a high-volume level-1 trauma center, the implementation of a scribe service increased the number of notes written per patient, filled in for notes that had previously been missed, and increased the capture of evaluation and management charges, all despite an overall downturn in patient volume during the study period.[34] Through the improved charge capture, scribes can be cost neutral or even net revenue generating additions to the clinical team. Although difficult to quantify, providers in the above study reported subjectively improved job satisfaction, and it is likely that the use of scribes may alleviate some of the EMR contributors to physician burnout.[34,39]

Speech recognition software provides another mechanism to improve EMR documentation efficiency. By creating text data from voice inputs, this technology theoretically would allow for quicker documentation, and could facilitate more timely documentation, with physicians documenting during rounds or even at bedside.[35] Most providers, however, use this technology in the same temporal fashion as manually entering text data (typically after patient encounters are concluded), and some have expressed hesitation about learning how to implement a new technology in an already busy clinical practice.[35] This technology has the potential to allow for active dictation of progress notes during rounds or while transferring between patients during rounds, improving clinician efficiency. Additional areas of active research include predictive dictation, using machine learning, which autocomplete in real time based on dictation history of the end user and clinical scenario.

FUTURE DIRECTIONS

As utilization of the EMR and clinical informatics increases in day-to-day practice, surgeons will play a central role as system users, data producers, and analyzers. Multidisciplinary efforts are underway to optimize the EMR for clinical use and research. Although recognizing the continued gaps between perceived and actual usability, the literature increasingly demonstrates the areas of streamlined EMR function as well as supplementary resources, including scribes and digital voice recognition, which promise the improved EMR usability and decreased EMR burden on clinicians.[41] To ensure that future EMR improvements meet the clinical needs of today's surgeon, surgical stakeholders should be proactive within their practices, health systems, professional groups, and in their legislative efforts to ensure that their needs are advocated for. These future directions include:

- Improved data entry: easier to input, easier to access, easier to analyze
- Improved access across health system with cross-platform interoperability
- More dynamic perioperative data gathering and processing to guide clinical decisions in real time

DISCUSSION
What Is the Electronic Medical Record to Today's Surgeon?

Although some of the topics touched on in this article may seem esoteric with questionable relevance to the day-to-day practice of surgeons across the country, they hopefully serve to demonstrate the many "hidden" facets of the EMR. Our interactions with electronic health records often feel limited to notes and orders between cases, electronic medication or laboratory orders, or a never-shrinking collection of inbox messages awaiting response. Yet, the EMR offers the possibility of actively shaping clinical care to be more efficient, effective, and safer. The preceding sections have highlighted the realms in which the EMR can and does shape the improved clinical practice. Health systems recognize this and invest time, energy, and financial resources into honing this tool to achieve better outcomes, decreased inefficiencies, and more dynamic data utilization. Surgeons can and should actively participate in this realm.

Most importantly, however, the EMR is beneficial to the people who surgeons center their entire careers on their patients. Whether through enabling predictive analytics to identify clinical deterioration early enough to intervene, optimizing surgical interventions to improve patient outcomes, or improving operating room flow to help more patients get the expeditious care they need, the EMR can be a critical tool for improving patient care.

SUMMARY

The EMR has undergone a substantial transformation over the past two decades and will continue to evolve in the future. The increasing amounts of tools and aids will be made accessible to the clinician through the EMR. However, knowledge of these systems and the implementation into clinical practice depends on the provider's willingness to use them. The ballooning of clinical data will continue to expand, and providers should take advantage of this resource to improve the care of patients.

It cannot be overstated that the conversion to EMRs over the past 30 years has dramatically transformed the way health care is delivered. It is important to recognize the shortcomings of the platform while also taking advantage of the underlying features to best benefit both the provider and the patient.

CLINICS CARE POINTS

- Electronic medical records can greatly benefit providers from their wealth of data but can also burden them with their documentation requirements.
- Real-time information within the electronic medical record can help guide decision suppport to provide superior care to patients.
- Data should be continuously reviewed within the electronic medical record as there is a tendency for erroneous data to propagate throughout the record system.

DISCLOSURE

No authors have received any financial benefit for participating in the development of this article. There are no conflicts of interest.

REFERENCES

1. Goldstein BA, Navar AM, Pencina MJ, et al. Opportunities and challenges in developing risk prediction models with electronic health records data: a systematic review. J Am Med Inform Assoc 2017-1;24(1):198–208.
2. Parasrampuria S, Henry J. Hospitals' Use of Electronic Health Records Data, 2015-2017. Available at: https://www.healthit.gov/sites/default/files/page/2019-04/AHAEHRUseDataBrief.pdf. Accessed July 3, 2022.
3. Maier-Hein L, Vedula S, Speidel S, et al. Surgical Data Science: Enabling next-generation surgery. :10.
4. Electronic Health Records. Available at: https://www.cms.gov/Medicare/E-Health/EHealthRecords. Accessed October 9, 2022.
5. Chodankar D. Introduction to real-world evidence studies. Perspect Clin Res 2021;12(3):171–4.
6. Davies A, Mueller J, Hassey A, et al. Development of a core competency framework for clinical informatics. BMJ Health Care Inform 2021;28(1):e100356.
7. Silverman HD, Steen EB, Carpenito JN, et al. Domains, tasks, and knowledge for clinical informatics subspecialty practice: results of a practice analysis. J Am Med Inform Assoc 2019;26(7):586–93.
8. Vedula SS, Hager GD. Surgical data science: the new knowledge domain. Innov Surg Sci 2017;2(3):109–21.
9. Rajkomar A, Dean J, Kohane I. Machine learning in medicine. N Engl J Med 2019;380(14):1347–58.
10. Churpek MM, Yuen TC, Park SY, et al. Using electronic health record data to develop and validate a prediction model for adverse outcomes in the wards. Crit Care Med 2014;42(4):841–8.
11. Bartkowiak B, Snyder AM, Benjamin A, et al. Validating the Electronic Cardiac Arrest Risk Triage (eCART) Score for Risk Stratification of Surgical Inpatients in the Postoperative Setting: Retrospective Cohort Study. Ann Surg 2019;269(6):1059–63.

12. Bartek MA, Saxena RC, Solomon S, et al. Improving operating room efficiency: machine learning approach to predict case-time duration. J Am Coll Surg 2019;229(4):346–54, e3.

13. Kothari AN, Brownlee SA, Blackwell RH, et al. Association between elements of electronic health record systems and the weekend effect in urgent general surgery. JAMA Surg 2017;152(6):602–3.

14. Martinez O, Martinez C, Parra CA, et al. Machine learning for surgical time prediction. Comput Methods Programs Biomed 2021;208:106220.

15. Tuwatananurak JP, Zadeh S, Xu X, et al. Machine learning can improve estimation of surgical case duration: a pilot study. J Med Syst 2019;43(3):44.

16. Huang L, Chen X, Liu W, et al. Automatic surgery and anesthesia emergence duration prediction using artificial neural networks. J Healthc Eng 2022;2022:2921775.

17. Collum TH, Menachemi N, Sen B. Does electronic health record use improve hospital financial performance? Evidence from panel data. Health Care Manage Rev 2016;41(3):267–74.

18. Howley MJ, Chou EY, Hansen N, et al. The long-term financial impact of electronic health record implementation. J Am Med Inform Assoc 2015;22(2):443–52.

19. Tsai CH, Eghdam A, Davoody N, et al. Effects of Electronic Health Record Implementation and Barriers to Adoption and Use: A Scoping Review and Qualitative Analysis of the Content. Life 2020;10(12). https://doi.org/10.3390/life10120327.

20. Sarangarm D, Lamb G, Weiss S, et al. Implementation of electronic charting is not associated with significant change in physician productivity in an academic emergency department. JAMIA Open 2018;1(2):227–32.

21. Beauvais B, Kruse CS, Fulton L, et al. Association of electronic health record vendors with hospital financial and quality performance: retrospective data analysis. J Med Internet Res 2021;23(4):e23961.

22. Wang T, Wang Y, McLeod A. Do health information technology investments impact hospital financial performance and productivity? Int J Account Inf Syst 2018;28:1–13.

23. Shervani S, Madden W, Gleason LJ. Electronic health record interoperability-why electronically discontinued medications are still dispensed. JAMA Intern Med 2021;181(10):1383–4.

24. Mukhiya SK, Lamo Y. An HL7 FHIR and GraphQL approach for interoperability between heterogeneous Electronic Health Record systems. Health Inform J 2021;27(3). 14604582211043920.

25. Negro-Calduch E, Azzopardi-Muscat N, Krishnamurthy RS, et al. Technological progress in electronic health record system optimization: systematic review of systematic literature reviews. Int J Med Inform 2021;152:104507.

26. Gianfrancesco MA, Tamang S, Yazdany J, et al. Potential biases in machine learning algorithms using electronic health record data. JAMA Intern Med 2018;178(11):1544–7.

27. Rajkomar A, Hardt M, Howell MD, et al. Ensuring fairness in machine learning to advance health equity. Ann Intern Med 2018;169(12):866–72.

28. Institute of Medicine (US) Committee on Understanding and Eliminating Racial and Ethnic Disparities in Health Care. Unequal Treatment: Confronting Racial and Ethnic Disparities in Health Care. Smedley BD, Stith AY, Nelson AR, editors. Washington (DC): National Academies Press (US); 2003. PMID: 25032386.

29. Department of Health and Human Services. Electronic medical records in healthcare. 2022. Available at: https://www.hhs.gov/sites/default/files/2022-02-17-1300-emr-in-healthcare-tlpwhite.pdf.

30. Fahy BG, Balke CW, Umberger GH, et al. Crossing the chasm: information technology to biomedical informatics. J Investig Med 2011-6;59(5):768–79.

31. Lee YL, Lee HA, Hsu CY, et al. SEMRES - a triple security protected blockchain based medical record exchange structure. Comput Methods Programs Biomed 2022;215:106595.

32. Chamola V, Goyal A, Sharma P, et al. Artificial intelligence-assisted blockchain-based framework for smart and secure EMR management. Neural Comput Appl 2022;1–11.

33. Shrivastava U, Song J, Han BT, et al. Do data security measures, privacy regulations, and communication standards impact the interoperability of patient health information? A cross-country investigation. Int J Med Inform 2021;148:104401.

34. Golob JF Jr, Como JJ, Claridge JA. Trauma surgeons save lives-scribes save trauma surgeons. Am Surg 2018;84(1):144–8.

35. Dymek C, Kim B, Melton GB, et al. Building the evidence-base to reduce electronic health record-related clinician burden. J Am Med Inform Assoc 2021; 28(5):1057–61.

36. Hobensack M, Levy DR, Cato K, et al. 25 × 5 Symposium to reduce documentation burden: report-out and call for action. Appl Clin Inform 2022;13(2):439–46.

37. Carayon P, Salwei ME. Moving toward a sociotechnical systems approach to continuous health information technology design: the path forward for improving electronic health record usability and reducing clinician burnout. J Am Med Inform Assoc 2021;28(5):1026–8.

38. Hettinger AZ, Melnick ER, Ratwani RM. Advancing electronic health record vendor usability maturity: Progress and next steps. J Am Med Inform Assoc 2021;28(5):1029–31.

39. Nguyen OT, Jenkins NJ, Khanna N, et al. A systematic review of contributing factors of and solutions to electronic health record-related impacts on physician well-being. J Am Med Inform Assoc 2021;28(5):974–84.

40. Sequeira L, Almilaji K, Strudwick G, et al. EHR "SWAT" teams: a physician engagement initiative to improve Electronic Health Record (EHR) experiences and mitigate possible causes of EHR-related burnout. JAMIA Open 2021;4(2): ooab018.

41. Poon EG, Trent Rosenbloom S, Zheng K. Health information technology and clinician burnout: Current understanding, emerging solutions, and future directions. J Am Med Inform Assoc 2021;28(5):895–8.

Modern Statistical Methods for the Surgeon Scientist
The Clash of Frequentist versus Bayesian Paradigms

Daniel Lammers, MD*, John McClellan, MD

KEYWORDS

- Statistics • Frequentist • Bayesian • Hypothesis

KEY POINTS

- Statistical methods remain an integral part of any study design; yet, a deep understanding of statistical design is often not part of medical training.
- Frequentist statistical methods remain the most commonly used techniques in the medical literature; however, they are often incorrectly interpreted.
- Bayesian statistics offer an alternative and more intuitive approach when assessing data.

INTRODUCTION

Evidence-based decision-making represents the guiding principle and standard of care within modern clinical practice.[1,2] Thus, a thorough and comprehensive understanding of the most up-to-date medical literature remains critical for surgeons. Furthermore, knowledge of the underlying study design and statistical techniques used within a protocol remain an integral key toward developing a true comprehension and mastery of the presented data. Although cursory statistical techniques are frequently taught throughout medical education, the statistical methods embedded within many clinical trials frequently extends beyond these basic tests. This often results in a multitude of hidden nuances within the outcomes not fully appreciated by the audience, commonly leading to the prevalent misuse and misinterpretation of even the most basic statistical results by medical researchers when describing clinical outcomes.[3–10]

By in large, the most common methodology for statistical inference centers on concepts such as P-values and confidence intervals in order to demonstrate significant

Department of General Surgery, Madigan Army Medical Center, 9040 Jackson Avenue, Tacoma, WA 98431, USA
* Corresponding author.
E-mail address: dtlammer@gmail.com

Surg Clin N Am 103 (2023) 259–269
https://doi.org/10.1016/j.suc.2022.12.001
0039-6109/23/Published by Elsevier Inc.

surgical.theclinics.com

associations between variables and outcomes in question. These concepts fall under a form of statistics referred to as frequentist statistics, which philosophically centers around the premise of rejecting a null hypothesis. Within medical and surgical trials, the null hypothesis traditionally states that there is no treatment effect between the groups being assessed. Therefore, a study is commonly referred to as being "successful" if the null hypothesis can be rejected. Rejection of the null hypothesis results from obtaining a final P-value that is less than the preset testing threshold. Briefly, P-values represent the probabilities that the outcome obtained, or one more extreme, will be present given that the null hypothesis is true.[11] The concepts surrounding P-values will be discussed in more detail in subsequent sections. Commonly though, the preconceived P-value threshold is set to .05, which corresponds to a Type I error rate of less than 5%. Despite this 5% Type I error rate threshold, the .05 P-value has recently come under attack as many statisticians and researchers think it represents an arbitrary cutoff that should be stricter (ie, $P < .005$) or even removed altogether.[12–16] This debate over P-values and their appropriate use, however, emphasizes a small portion of the controversies and limitations commonly discussed surrounding null-hypothesis significance testing that remains unbeknownst to most clinicians.

In this article, we intend to highlight the underlying workings of frequentist statistics while providing an in-depth look into their benefits and limitations. Moreover, we will explore Bayesian statistics, an alternative statistical framework that centers around deriving probability estimates associated with a hypothesis or treatment effect in question. Frequentist and Bayesian approaches will be compared in order to demonstrate key differences between the approaches. Finally, we will evaluate these statistical approaches in the context of a recent clinical study to highlight how each of these techniques can shape the outcomes of a trial.

Frequentist Statistics—Frequently Used but Frequently Misunderstood

Frequentist approaches, which remain the predominate form of statistics used in medical research, hinge on the assumption that the sample outcomes will ultimately occur at a set frequency or rate if infinite repeated sampling were to occur.[17] This approach assumes that the evaluated data is just one of many hypothetical data sets addressing the same question. This notion that an outcome frequency or rate occurs during the course of infinite hypothetical data sets, despite the performed research typically only obtaining a single data set, provides the structural basis for the frequentist approach.[18] Frequentists view a model (ie, a data set) as variable and the outcomes as unknown entities that should remain consistent or fixed.[19,20] Although each model will naturally display a degree of differences based on the samples included in the data set, the frequentist framework accounts for these variabilities based on sampling error and chance. These concepts explain why 2 equally designed experiments may obtain different results.[20]

At its philosophic core, the frequentist approach suggests that as the number of trials increases, the observed relative frequency of the event in question will get closer to that event's "true" value. Thus, when evaluating a treatment effect using a frequentist mindset, there will always be a true, yet unknown, value that the data is eventually poised to obtain if given the appropriate time to accrue enough data. The observed outcomes will become increasingly close to the true value as sample size increases or with additional iterative trials, depending on the study design. For instance, let us assess a scenario where a researcher flips a standard coin 10 times with the coin landing on heads 7 times and tails 3 times. Despite displaying a 70% prevalence of heads based on the last 10 coin flips, a frequentist observer would say that this trial is just one small representative sample of an infinite number of potential trials. Due to the infinite hypothetical samples, the small observed sample size has the potential for a high degree of error. Intuitively, it would make sense for the observer to suggest the true rate of obtaining heads is 50% (assuming they believed the coin was fair) and the discrepancy was secondary to error. Because of this, the true rate of obtaining heads before flipping the coin will eventually be uncovered with more data accumulation. The frequentist belief suggests that if someone were to flip the coin 10,000 times, roughly 5000 trials would result in heads and 5000 would result in tails. That said, due to error and chance, these values may be 4000 heads and 6000 tails. However, as the number of times the coin is flipped approaches infinity, a frequentist would expect to see the rate of heads being exactly 50% of the trials because this represents the true rate associated with each flip.

Conversely, what if the researcher were to flip the coin again and ask, "*What is the chance the coin landed on heads?*" A pure frequentist observer would not answer 50% (or even 70% based on the prevalence from the first 10 flips). In fact, they would view this question as discordant with their beliefs and suggest that because the coin has already landed, it is either 100% heads or 0% heads. By frequentist standards, the true value is fixed within a population and does not vary; only the data surrounding it does. As the models encompassing these values within this paradigm remain fluid, accounting for observed variances between sample sizes and various trials (as demonstrated with the hypothetical coin toss resulting in 7 heads) allows researchers the opportunity to present data in a way that is comparable during a series of experiments. Although there can be reported variance and error surrounding the frequentist's true value, there are no probabilities associated with the true values. The outcomes are reported with 100% certainty, as the goal of frequentist statistics is to highlight the unknown true value. Thus, the value either *is* or *is not*. Posing statements such as, "we believe our results are 50% probable," remains nonsensical under this statistical framework because there is not a range of possible outcomes within this philosophy, only a single true value.

As previously stated, frequentist statistics focus largely on null-hypothesis testing. The identification and accurate understanding of hypotheses remain critical to understanding this approach. During this process, one starts with a clinical question in mind and derives a null hypothesis. The null hypothesis suggests that there is no identifiable difference between the groups being assessed for the outcome in question. This offers the statistical basis for evaluation via the *P*-values obtained. *P*-values represent the probability of observing the outcome obtained, or one more extreme, if the null hypothesis is true. *P*-values, by definition, cannot provide direct evidence in favor of treatment effects. Instead, they can only allow researchers to simply reject the null hypothesis.[11] Using these approaches there is, however, no possible way to statistically prove a treatment effect is present.[10,21] As such, these concepts are convoluted and lead to frequent misinterpretations within the surgical literature.[3,4,10,11,14] In nontechnical language, one must assume going into the study that there is no difference between study cohorts. Then, based on the outcomes and results, decide how surprised they were by the outcomes. If there is a low probability (ie, low *P*-value) that the outcomes observed could be represented by the preconceived notion that there is no difference between the groups, the researcher's findings would be surprising. This would allow them to infer that the null hypothesis does not adequately explain the data observed and an outside factor (ie, the treatment in question) may account for the difference. The probability associated with the *P*-value, however, should not be confused with the desired true value of the treatment effect because these are 2 different entities. As such, the *P*-value does not tell the reader how true a hypothesis is, the magnitude, or size a treatment effect displays.[10,11] Because these statistical methods only offer an indirect approach toward endorsing a treatment effect, they fail to reflect the actual ability to prove that an alternative hypothesis is in fact true.[11] These concepts are often viewed as convoluted and remain misunderstood by many.[3] Despite this inability to directly prove differences between cohorts and their associated misinterpretations, these techniques remain the most commonly taught and used methods within medical statistics.

For example, let us assess a new pharmacologic being designed to decrease mortality from a certain disease process. In order to evaluate this novel drug, 2 groups of patients with the disease are randomized to either receive the drug intervention or a placebo. At the conclusion of the study, it is found that the absolute mortality was decreased within the cohort that took the study drug. However, under the frequentist paradigm, assessment of the associated P-value is now required to better understand and classify these findings. Assuming a P-value of .03 was obtained, what conclusions could be made? Other than stating that this is a statistically significant value based on a traditional P-threshold of .05, this value describes a 3% probability of observing the same or greater mortality difference described within the study in a world where the null hypothesis (ie, no mortality difference) is actually true. Due to this low value, the null hypothesis can be rejected because the actual mortality difference observed has a low enough probability of being represented under the null hypothesis. What if the P-value was .3? This would indicate that there is a 30% chance of observing the same or greater mortality difference in a world where there was no true difference. Statistically speaking, the risk of an associated Type I error is too high in this scenario and represents an instance where we would not be able to reject the null hypothesis. This remains conceptually challenging to nonstatisticians and brings forth a model poised for misunderstanding. Because the P-value represents a probability associated with rejecting the null hypothesis, not the probability associated with the outcome in question, it remains a commonly misunderstood value. Thus, as previously discussed, the frequentist's outcome should have no probability value tethered it. Yet, due to the convoluted and indirect association between outcomes and P-values, this approach remains challenging for many.[3,10,11]

Although P-values alone do not provide information regarding the size of the effect, confidence intervals can help provide deeper insight into the magnitude and direction of an effect size between study cohorts. The size of the confidence interval chosen, which traditionally is set to 95%, illustrates that the true mean or frequency would be found within this reported range 95% (or whatever threshold is decided on) of the time if the experiment were to be run over a series of infinitely repeated trials.[22] Naturally, wider confidence intervals represent models with more uncertainty. Due to this, statisticians urge that readers should view confidence intervals more stringently when assessing clinical trials that contain statistically significant results before determining their final conclusion. For instance, using the mortality reduction example previously described during the P-value discussion, assume a study found a mortality difference of 10% ($P = .03$) associated with a novel drug. A 95% confidence interval ranging from 8% to 11% provides a much more precise estimate than a 95% confidence interval ranging from 1% to 19%. It is important to note, however, that a 95% confidence interval does not tell us that there is a 95% chance that the true value can be found within this interval. This concept, similar to P-values, poses a difficult concept to grasp. However, this is consistent with the general theory behind frequentist statistics, which state that because there is only one true outcome, assigning a probability to that specific outcome (ie, 95% probability that the value is within the interval) is not conceptually valid. The confidence interval, therefore, should be viewed as a range of values from a fictitious population of experiments repeated numerous times and does not represent a one-time snapshot of the actual data observed. Thus, using frequentist methods, the true value should be considered either 100% within or 100% outside the associated confidence interval.

BAYESIAN STATISTICS—PROBABILITIES OF OUTCOMES PROVIDE OPPORTUNITIES FOR INTUITIVE RESULTS

Alternatively, Bayesian statistics represent a fundamentally different statistical approach based on assigning a probability distribution toward a specific hypothesis. With this approach, the data and model are viewed as a fixed entity with probabilities assigned to variable possible outcomes based on the observed data. Bayesian techniques represent a direct contrast to the frequentist approach and the belief of a universally fixed outcome. This approach provides uncertainty within the outcome, as opposed to the uncertainty being allocated to the data.[23–27] Continuing with the previous discussions surrounding a 10% absolute mortality difference with the use of a novel drug, a Bayesian approach would be able to make a claim such as there being a 98% probability that mortality is improved by at least 10% with this new drug compared with a placebo based on the data observed within the trial. This concept is thought to be more intuitive because it only assesses the data that has been obtained and does not consider a multitude of hypothetical data points.

Moreover, because Bayesian approaches focus on the probabilities of outcomes, these probabilities can be updated without penalty as more data are collected.[28] Interestingly, when more data are collected, the Bayesian process allows one to use the previously collected information that was known before the newly acquired data was obtained (termed "prior") and performs an iterative adjustment to the previously accepted outcome. This provides the most possible updated results that are directly based only on the total data assessed. Although it makes logical sense to use priors during continuous data collection, a main benefit of this approach is the ability to use data from similarly designed previously performed studies to help provide a starting framework for the newly acquired data to update. Using priors in this fashion offers the ability to decrease sample sizes while still obtaining meaningful results.[25,29,30] When combined, the collective prior and newly used data yield the most updated results referred to as the posterior distribution.

Because the utilization of prior information can help influence the results, Bayesian skeptics argue that this effect brings forth the potential for undue bias.[31] Just as with any study, transparency on how the selected prior was obtained remains a critical component to assure reproducibility of results.[32,33] That said, in order to mitigate the risk for potential bias, strategies focusing on a multiplicity of alternative priors have been used.[34] These include using noninformative priors, as well as incorporating multiple priors that span a wide array of assumptions. Noninformative priors provide no additional information to the model and are regarded as neutral. Therefore, the posterior probability obtained when using a noninformative prior is strictly reliant on the observed data.[35–37] Imputation of numerous priors during the course of multiple models represents an interesting approach that results in an array of outcomes influenced by priors ranging from skeptical to optimistic treatment effects. This approach allows researchers the ability to observe how study results could be influenced over a spectrum of potential clinical scenarios.[37]

Further, Bayesian approaches can be used to calculate the probabilities of specific hypotheses with respect to others. For instance, using Bayesian statistics one can directly calculate the probability that treatment A is superior to treatment B. This allows for statistical evidence that one treatment is superior to another, which, as described previously, is not possible using frequentist approaches.[38] Moreover, not only can one demonstrate superiority, a degree of certainty can be placed on the results leading to more granular data (ie, there is a 98% chance that treatment A is superior to treatment B). These degrees of certainty can be further represented by performing threshold analyses between 2 hypotheses.[39,40] For instance, not only can one ascertain that there is a 98% chance that treatment A is superior to treatment B (ie, RR < 1), one can make claims such as there is a 75% chance that treatment A offers at least a 30% reduction in the outcome assessed compared with treatment B (ie, RR < 0.7). As evident here, Bayesian approaches do not yield a P-value. Therefore, when interpreting these results, one must be cognizant of this change in paradigm. Bayesian approaches do, however, allow for the derivation of Bayes factors. Bayes factors provide an alternative measurement that is able to quantify support for one model over another. This is done by calculating a likelihood ratio between the 2 competing hypotheses based on the data obtained.[38] The 2 hypotheses in question can represent a null hypothesis and an alternative, similar to that of frequentist statistics; however, they are not limited to these and can represent any hypothesis desired. As Bayes factors represent a comparative ratio, the values range from zero to infinity with more extreme values providing stronger evidence in support of the studied hypothesis.

Just as frequentist approaches provide the potential for confidence intervals, Bayesian approaches offer the ability to calculate the highest density interval (HDI).[25] Similar to confidence intervals, HDI often has an associated 95% with it. Despite the attachment of a similar numeric value, HDI represents a conceptually different value compared with the frequentist confidence interval. A 95% HDI states that over the probability distribution from the data observed, 95% of the most probable values will be included in this range. This differs from a 95% confidence interval because it only directly assesses the data that was observed and provides a probability that the treatment effect can be found within this range. A wide HDI, similar to wide confidence intervals, represents a scenario with more uncertainty surrounding the data. As such, confidence intervals and HDI pose ranges of values that differ due to the divergent fundamental concepts associated with frequentist and Bayesian statistics.

Clashing Paradigms—a Case Example via a Modern Clinical Trial

As demonstrated above, frequentist and Bayesian methods approach a clinical question from 2 different viewpoints that allow for different answers. Although one statistical approach is not necessarily better or worse than the other, understanding the limitations of each allows for the best statistical analysis to be performed. Recently, many frequentist trials have been reevaluated using Bayesian approaches to highlight these differences and bring awareness to Bayesian approaches. Often, however, these contrasting viewpoints lead to differing conclusions and further drive the divide between traditional frequentist and Bayesian statisticians.

To highlight these concepts, the use of extracorporeal membrane oxygenation (ECMO) for severe acute respiratory distress syndrome (ARDS) represents a relevant clinical example. ECMO represents an invasive approach to provide respiratory and cardiac support for critically ill patients by diverting blood flow from their cardiopulmonary system into a heart-lung machine in order to promote gas exchange and improve perfusion. The ECMO to Rescue Lung Injury in Severe ARDS (EOLIA) trial was an international clinical trial that randomly assigned patients with severe ARDS to receive either venovenous ECMO or continue with conventional therapy through standard ventilator support, prone positioning, and neuromuscular blockade. EOLIA was designed under a frequentist paradigm to assess 60-day mortality using a group sequential analysis that allowed for early stopping based on perceived demonstration of superiority, harm, or a predicted lack of difference. The study was initially designed to demonstrate a 20% mortality reduction in the ECMO cohort (60% vs 40%). Due to the prespecified stopping rules set during the design process, the study was stopped after 240 patients despite being originally designed for a maximum of 331 participants, based on 80% power and alpha level of 5%. Early stopping was a result of a failure to perceive a significant difference in 60-day mortality as evidenced by a 35% mortality in the ECMO cohort and 46% in the control (RR = 0.76; 95% CI = 0.55–1.04; P = .09) at this time period. Based on these findings, the authors concluded that ECMO was not associated with a significantly lower mortality rate compared with the control group.[41] As such, they failed to reject their null hypothesis, and this trial was seen on the surface as a "negative trial."

Recognizing the limitations of the EOLIA trial, Goligher and colleagues performed a Bayesian post hoc analysis to demonstrate the potential utility of these methods for assessing clinical trials. Limitations of the original EOLIA trial included early stopping following reaching only 75% of the maximum sample size and a high crossover rate. As the original study was powered to detect a 20% absolute risk difference, it was thought to be underpowered, especially as the 11% absolute mortality reduction displayed a perceived clinically significant result. This Bayesian reanalysis estimated the posterior probabilities that ECMO demonstrated a treatment effect over a range of values with the goal to identify the most clinically important values. This was performed using noninformative priors, as well a variety of plausible priors ranging from strongly enthusiastic to strongly skeptical, in order to highlight a range of possibilities surrounding the preexisting controversy over ECMO and its use. From this analysis, the authors were able to demonstrate that there was at least an 88% probability that ECMO was superior to conventional ventilator strategies with regards to 60-day mortality based on the range of priors assessed. Further, depending on the prior data used, a 78% to 98% probability of displaying at least a 2% absolute mortality reduction (the minimal clinically relevant value) was found.[34]

Through this Bayesian reanalysis, the authors were able to provide evidence in support of a mortality benefit using ECMO for severe ARDS under a broad set of clinical assumptions. The conclusions drawn from the original EOLIA trial differ due to the framework surrounding the original questions being asked. EOLIA attempted to estimate the probability of the data given the hypothesis (ie, provide evidence against the null-hypothesis), whereas the Bayesian counterpart estimated the probabilities of the hypothesis given the observed data. Although these differing viewpoints may seem trivial on the surface, the EOLIA trial and this associated Bayesian post hoc analysis demonstrate the potential conflicting nature of these 2 approaches and the clinical implications associated with each.

DISCUSSION AND LIMITATIONS

Bayesian and frequentist schools of thought contrast each other in the way they view clinical problems. However, this does not mean that one should solely focus on one approach as opposed to the other. In fact, both display unique benefits when interpreted correctly and they can be used to support and bolster one another clinically. With regards to study design, having a predesigned statistical plan remains critical because it will help ensure appropriate methods are being implemented to obtain the best quality of data. Although frequentist approaches have dominated the realm of clinical trial design, the improvements in computational software to include

Bayesian techniques into many standard statistical packages have allowed for improved ease of use and access by researchers seeking Bayesian methods.[26]

Although the potential for subjective bias based on prior elicitation remains possible with Bayesian approaches, techniques such as incorporation of multiple priors or non-informative priors can help to overcome these subjective biases and result in outcomes congruent with our natural approach of reasoning.[34] Frequentist approaches, however, are not immune to subjective bias as manipulation of the data or alteration of the prespecified study design can result in artificially derived statistical significance, a term commonly referred to as P hacking.[42,43] Ultimately, transparency within the statistical approach and trial methods to allow for clinical reproducibility remains critical for proper study design.

Sample size determination has traditionally been an important element of trial design under the frequentist approach. This should be carefully calculated as incorrect sample sizes can lead to inconclusive results or wasted resources.[44–46] Sample size formulation is done following the determination of the expected treatment effect, Type I error rate, Type II error rate, and baseline control rate. Traditionally, clinical trials have used a Type I error rate of 5% (corresponding to an alpha values of 0.05) and Type II error rate of 20% (corresponding to a beta value of 80%). Based on the associated calculations, scenarios where the treatment effect is small will ultimately result in extremely large sample sizes. Although robust patient populations may be easy to obtain for various prevalent disease processes, rare pathologic conditions (ie, congenital disorders) or processes with highly variable populations (ie, trauma) may be difficult recruit suitable study populations and result in the potential for poor data quality.[47] Bayesian approaches, however, do not technically require sample size estimates before the study. Due to their ability to allow for sequential learning without penalty, Bayesian approaches readily lend themselves to these populations, whereas frequentist properties are affected by the number and timing of interim analyses. As such, Bayesian approaches can continuously assess their data and terminate the study when sufficient data have been obtained. This offers the potential for significantly smaller sample sizes compared with traditional frequentist designs.[23,29,30] Bayesian trial design may, therefore, be more appropriate for traditionally difficult patient populations to study.

Regardless of choosing a frequentist or Bayesian approach, it is essential to remember that the statistical methods chosen for the analysis will neither overcome poor study design nor combat poor data quality. Thus, stringent adherence to the proper principles of trial design remains necessary. Efforts focusing on patient recruitment, randomization, blinding (if possible), and appropriate control groups need to be an early focus from the research team. Further, assuring the selected endpoints appropriately reflect the study question remains a critical, yet often overlooked, portion of the study design. For instance, trauma studies evaluating hemorrhagic shock traditionally used 24-hour and 30-day mortality as their endpoints. Physiologic data, however, suggests that most patients who die from hemorrhagic shock will do so within the first 6 hours. Therefore, assessing 24-hour and 30-day mortality to evaluate how a specific treatment alters hemorrhage-associated mortality does not optimally reflect the intended purpose.[48,49] These strategies and principles remain critical components for effective trial design.

SUMMARY

In conclusion, evidence-based medicine is critical to assuring optimal patient care. Evidence, however, remain widely variable within the medical literature. Although knowing the outcomes from clinical trials remains critically important, understanding how those outcomes were obtained should hold equal, if not more, importance. Although frequentist and Bayesian schools of thought differ in their approaches to how they view clinical problems, both provide valid options for trial design. Regardless of the approach used, the correct interpretation of the statistics is required. Although frequentist approaches have traditionally dominated clinical trials, Bayesian techniques are becoming increasingly more popular due to the inherent flexibility they provide. Due to this, improved educational awareness of medical statistics, both frequentist and Bayesian, should be more formally incorporated into medical training to ensure future generations of surgeon scientists have the necessary tools to answer the most pressing clinical questions.

CLINICS CARE POINTS

- Bayesian statistics revolve around probabilities between competing hypotheses.
- Bayesian approaches can provide evidence in support of the alternative hypothesis, whereas frequentist statistics cannot.
- Frequentists statistics often result in a false dichotomization based on an arbitrary P-value.

DISCLOSURE

The authors have nothing to disclose.

REFERENCES

1. Guyatt G, Cairns J, Churchill D, et al. Evidence-based medicine: a new approach to teaching the practice of medicine. Jama 1992;268(17):2420–5.
2. Timmermans S, Berg M. The gold standard: the challenge of evidence-based medicine. Philadelphia: Temple University Press; 2010.
3. Windish DM, Huot SJ, Green ML. Medicine Residents' Understanding of the Biostatistics and Results in the Medical Literature. JAMA 2007;298(9):1010–22.
4. Thiese MS, Ronna B, Robbins RB. Misuse of statistics in surgical literature. J Thorac Dis 2016;8(8):E726–30.
5. Colquhoun D. An investigation of the false discovery rate and the misinterpretation of p-values. R Soc Open Sci 2014;1(3):140216.
6. Colquhoun D. The reproducibility of research and the misinterpretation of p-values. R Soc Open Sci 2017;4(12):171085.
7. Greenland S, Senn SJ, Rothman KJ, et al. Statistical tests, P values, confidence intervals, and power: a guide to misinterpretations. Eur J Epidemiol 2016;31(4): 337–50.
8. Hoekstra R, Morey RD, Rouder JN, et al. Robust misinterpretation of confidence intervals. Psychon Bull Rev 2014;21(5):1157–64.
9. Ioannidis JPA. Why Most Published Research Findings Are False. PLOS Med 2005;2(8):e124.
10. Goodman S. A Dirty Dozen: Twelve P-Value Misconceptions. Semin Hematol 2008;45(3):135–40.
11. Wasserstein RL, Lazar NA. The ASA Statement on p-Values: Context, Process, and Purpose. Am Stat 2016;70(2):129–33.

12. Amrhein V, Greenland S, McShane B. Scientists rise up against statistical significance. Nature 2019;567(7748):305–7.
13. Ioannidis JP. The proposal to lower P value thresholds to. 005. Jama 2018; 319(14):1429–30.
14. Betensky RA. The p-value requires context, not a threshold. Am Stat 2019; 73(sup1):115–7.
15. Benjamin DJ, Berger JO, Johannesson M, et al. Redefine statistical significance. Nat Hum Behav 2018;2(1):6–10.
16. Kraemer HC. Is It time to ban the p value? JAMA Psychiatry 2019;76(12): 1219–20.
17. Howson C, Urbach P. Scientific reasoning: the bayesian approach. Chicao and La Salle (IL): Open Court Publishing; 2006. p. 344.
18. Goodman SN. Toward evidence-based medical statistics. 1: the p value fallacy. Ann Intern Med 1999;130(12):995–1004.
19. Bland JM, Altman DG. Bayesians and frequentists. BMJ 1998;317(7166): 1151–60.
20. Samaniego FJ. A comparison of the Bayesian and frequentist approaches to estimation, 24. New York: Springer; 2010.
21. Neyman J, Pearson ES, IX. On the problem of the most efficient tests of statistical hypotheses. Philos Trans R Soc Lond Ser Contain Pap Math Phys Character 1933;231(694–706):289–337.
22. Berger JO, Wolpert RL. The likelihood principle. Hayward (CA): IMS; 1988. p. 262.
23. Hampson LV, Whitehead J, Eleftheriou D, et al. Bayesian methods for the design and interpretation of clinical trials in very rare diseases. Stat Med 2014;33(24): 4186–201.
24. Gelman A, Shalizi CR. Philosophy and the practice of Bayesian statistics. Br J Math Stat Psychol 2013;66(1):8–38.
25. Bolstad WM, Curran JM. Introduction to bayesian statistics. Hoboken (NJ): John Wiley & Sons; 2016.
26. van de Schoot R, Depaoli S, King R, et al. Bayesian statistics and modelling. Nat Rev Methods Primer 2021;1(1):1–26.
27. Lilford RJ, Thornton JG, Braunholtz D. Clinical trials and rare diseases: a way out of a conundrum. BMJ 1995;311(7020):1621–5.
28. Gelman A, Hill J, Yajima M. Why we (usually) don't have to worry about multiple comparisons. J Res Educ Eff 2012;5(2):189–211.
29. Jansen JO, Pallmann P, MacLennan G, et al. Investigators the URT. Bayesian clinical trial designs: Another option for trauma trials? J Trauma Acute Care Surg 2017;83(4):736–41.
30. Gsponer T, Gerber F, Bornkamp B, et al. A practical guide to Bayesian group sequential designs. Pharm Stat 2014;13(1):71–80.
31. Van Dongen S. Prior specification in bayesian statistics: three cautionary tales. J Theor Biol 2006;242(1):90–100.
32. Kruschke JK. Bayesian Analysis Reporting Guidelines. Nat Hum Behav 2021; 5(10):1282–91.
33. van Doorn J, van den Bergh D, Böhm U, et al. The JASP guidelines for conducting and reporting a Bayesian analysis. Psychon Bull Rev 2021;28(3):813–26.
34. Goligher EC, Tomlinson G, Hajage D, et al. Extracorporeal membrane oxygenation for severe acute respiratory distress syndrome and posterior probability of mortality benefit in a post hoc Bayesian analysis of a randomized clinical trial. JAMA 2018;320(21):2251–9.

35. Kass RE, Wasserman L. The selection of prior distributions by formal rules. J Am Stat Assoc 1996;91(435):1343–70.
36. Ghosh M. Objective priors: an introduction for frequentists. Stat Sci 2011;26(2): 187–202.
37. Fayers PM, Ashby D, Parmar MKB. Tutorial in biostatistics: bayesian data monitoring in clinical trials. Stat Med 1997;16(12):1413–30.
38. Kass RE, Raftery AE. Bayes factors. J Am Stat Assoc 1995;90(430):773–95.
39. Diamond GA, Kaul S. Prior convictions. J Am Coll Cardiol 2004;43(11):1929–39.
40. Harrell FE, Shih YC. Using full probability models to compute probabilities of actual interest to decision makers. Int J Technol Assess Health Care 2001; 17(1):17–26.
41. Combes A, Hajage D, Capellier G, et al. Extracorporeal membrane oxygenation for severe acute respiratory distress syndrome. N Engl J Med 2018;378(21): 1965–75.
42. Adda J, Decker C, Ottaviani M. P-hacking in clinical trials and how incentives shape the distribution of results across phases. Proc Natl Acad Sci 2020; 117(24):13386–92.
43. Head ML, Holman L, Lanfear R, et al. The extent and consequences of p-hacking in science. Plos Biol 2015;13(3):e1002106.
44. Altman DG. Statistics and ethics in medical research: III How large a sample? Br Med J 1980;281(6251):1336–8.
45. Freiman JA, Chalmers TC, Smith HA, et al. The Importance of Beta, the Type II Error, and Sample Size in the Design and Interpretation of the Randomized Controlled Trial: Survey of Two Sets of "Negative" Trials. In: Medical uses of statistics. 2nd edition. Boca Raton (FL): CRC Press; 1992. p. 357–89.
46. Moher D, Dulberg CS, Wells GA. Statistical power, sample size, and their reporting in randomized controlled trials. JAMA 1994;272(2):122–4.
47. Abrahamyan L, Feldman BM, Tomlinson G, et al. Alternative designs for clinical trials in rare diseases. Am J Med Genet C Semin Med Genet 2016;172(4):313–31.
48. Fox EE, Holcomb JB, Wade CE, et al, PROPPR Study Group. Earlier endpoints are required for hemorrhagic shock trials among severely injured patients. Shock Augusta Ga 2017;47(5):567–73.
49. Holcomb JB, Moore EE, Sperry JL, et al. Evidence-based and clinically relevant outcomes for hemorrhage control trauma trials. Ann Surg 2021;273(3):395–401.

Cognitive Bias and Dissonance in Surgical Practice: A Narrative Review

Caroline E. Richburg, BS[a], Lesly A. Dossett, MD, MPH[b],
Tasha M. Hughes, MD, MPH[b],*

KEYWORDS

- Cognitive bias • Heuristics • Cognitive dissonance • Decision-making
- Surgical error

KEY POINTS

- A cognitive bias describes "shortcuts" subconsciously applied to new scenarios to simplify decision-making. In some cases, this can lead to error in medical decision-making.
- Cognitive biases in surgery have been shown to result in delayed surgical intervention, unnecessary procedures, intraoperative error, and delayed recognition of postoperative complications.
- "Metacognition," or pausing to think about the way we think, is an evidence-based strategy to reduce cognitive bias in clinical practice.

INTRODUCTION

A 45-year-old mother of three with a past medical history significant for obesity presents with several months of intermittent right upper quadrant pain that has now become constant and more severe. *Cholelithiasis*, you're thinking, expecting a laparoscopic cholecystectomy on your schedule soon. This automatic, largely unconscious line of reasoning that allows you jump to a diagnosis based on relatively small amounts of data is referred to as "fast" or "system one" thinking. This pathway of thinking is in stark contrast to "system two" or "slow" thinking, which is deliberate, analytical, and effortful.[1,2] Nobel Prize winner Daniel Kahneman describes in his book, *Thinking Fast and Slow*, that even when system one thinking dominates "most of our judgements

[a] University of Michigan Medical School, 1500 East Medical Center Drive, Ann Arbor, MI, USA;
[b] Department of Surgery, Michigan Medicine, 2101 Taubman Center, 1500 East Medical Center Drive, Ann Arbor, MI, USA
* Corresponding author. Rogel Cancer Center Spc 3294, 1500 E Medical Center Drive, Ann Arbor, MI 48109.
E-mail address: tmhughes@med.umich.edu
Twitter: @cerichburg (C.E.R.); @leslydossett (L.A.D.); @tashahughesmd (T.M.H.)

Surg Clin N Am 103 (2023) 271–285
https://doi.org/10.1016/j.suc.2022.11.003
0039-6109/23/© 2022 Elsevier Inc. All rights reserved.

surgical.theclinics.com

and actions are appropriate most of the time,"[1] and so goes the old trope, "when you hear hooves, think horses, not zebras." Such reasoning and decisive action are particularly relevant in surgery. Although there are many situations where action based on this quick system of thinking is necessary and even lifesaving, such thought processes are also susceptible to the unintentional and often unrecognized introduction of cognitive bias.[3] For instance, with our patient presumed to have cholelithiasis, the consulting surgeon may cease diagnostic evaluation and miss that the patient instead has a rare hemorrhagic hepatic adenoma, perforated ulcer, or other less common diagnosis.[4] This potential for missed diagnosis is the consequence of cognitive bias in action.

A cognitive bias describes "shortcuts" (ie, "heuristics") which are subconsciously applied to new situations to simplify decision-making, such as in our case where right upper quadrant pain in an obese woman of child-bearing age is presumed, possibly prematurely, to represent cholelithiasis.[5] **Table 1** summarizes a list of cognitive biases most relevant in the care of surgical patients with definitions and clinically relevant examples. A cognitive bias is distinct from implicit bias, which describes unconscious assumptions based on race, gender, sexual orientation, age, and other identities. For example, if we assumed that because our patient presenting with right upper quadrant pain is a woman and therefore is weak and cannot tolerate pain as well as a male patient, we would be introducing implicit bias in the same clinical scenario. Although implicit biases are important and warrant research and attention in surgical practice, the following review focuses on cognitive bias in surgery and highlighting ways to minimize its effects through intentional "debiasing" efforts.

Nature of the Problem

Data generated from the internal medicine and emergency medicine literature suggest that a significant amount of diagnostic errors made in medicine occur secondary to the introduction of cognitive bias.[6] These same data suggest that error due to cognitive biases is not a rare occurrence, but rather one that impacts patient care on a regular basis.[6] Other studies have examined cognitive bias in the context of clinical decision-making more broadly than just diagnostic errors. A recent review of the cognitive bias literature found that most studies focused on hypothetical clinical scenarios posed to study participants and that only a minority of studies directly investigated real-life patient care, suggesting a gap in research.[7]

Although not as robust as other fields, there is a small body of work characterizing the role of cognitive biases specifically in surgery. The relative paucity of research in surgery likely reflects a historical gap in social and human behavior research within the surgical disciplines. Surgical decision-making happens quickly in a variety of settings including the emergency department (ED), the operating room, and the intensive care unit, with potential cognitive bias across each of these care settings. In this review, the authors aim to characterize the available literature on cognitive biases in surgery across all phases of care, from the diagnosis of surgical disease to care of the postoperative patient, with an attempt to highlight the best available research, identify gaps in the current surgical literature, and introduce possible strategies that have been proposed to mitigate the impact of cognitive bias in health care delivery.

DISCUSSION
The Prevalence of Cognitive Bias Across the Surgical Care Spectrum

Given that up to 74% of diagnostic error in internal medicine may be attributed to cognitive biases, we assume that the unintended introduction of these biases has a

Table 1
Common cognitive biases

Cognitive Bias	Clinically Focused Definition	Clinically Relevant Example
Base-rate neglect	Tendency to overestimate how common or uncommon a finding or diagnosis is within a general population when viewing an individual case	A surgeon overestimates the prevalence of an uncommon disease in interpreting test results[8]
Confirmation bias	Tendency to look for data that confirm one's prior beliefs	Looking for gallbladder findings on CT to support a presumed diagnosis of cholangitis at the expense of other findings[25]
Anchoring bias	Tendency to base clinical decisions on the first piece of diagnostic information	Comorbid patient presenting with orthopnea is diagnosed with CHF[19]
Escalation of commitment	Continued investment of resources despite evidence of impending failure[40]	Repeated abdominal washouts and reoperations despite clinical deterioration with poor prognosis[40]
Availability bias	Tendency to assess the likelihood of an event or diagnosis based on what instances or diagnoses come to mind	Misdiagnosis of acute hypoxic respiratory failure as COVID amidst pandemic despite negative testing[17]
Commission bias	Tendency to choose action over inaction[7]	Treating a low-grade cancer that is not expected to harm the patient[13]
Default bias	Tendency to keep the status quo[7]	Repeatedly diagnosing COVID during the COVID-19 pandemic
Optimism bias	Tendency to believe that an outcome will be positive	A surgeon who believes their anastomotic leak rate is lower than average does not form diverting stoma because they expect no leak[31]
Order effects: primacy and recency	Information presented at the beginning or end of a series is used more than that in the middle[7]	A patient's presenting symptoms are fever and dyspnea. Despite a full history, these presenting findings elicit a diagnosis of pneumonia[27]
Diagnostic momentum	An incorrect diagnosis made by a previous clinician is not questioned	Treatment of "pneumonia" did not improve patient's volume overload. Instead of questioning initial diagnosis, volume overload was misattributed to a dialysis catheter[18]

(continued on next page)

Table 1
(continued)

Cognitive Bias	Clinically Focused Definition	Clinically Relevant Example
Framing effect	Decisions are influenced by the way that information is presented	A patient presents to cardiomyopathy clinic with a misdiagnosis of "suspected cardiomyopathy"[20]
Overconfidence bias	Belief that one is better than average	Surgeons who believe they have a better-than-average anastomotic leak rate are less likely to form diverting loops[31]
Recall bias	Inaccurate, inconsistent, or incomplete recollection of an event	Surgical team is universally inaccurate in recounting major operating room events 1 week postoperation[35]
Visual misperception	"Seeing what you believe"[29]	Most laparoscopic bile duct injuries are secondary to misidentification of the duct[29]
Left-digit bias	The left-most digit in a variable tends to categorize the whole variable	An 80-year-old patient is perceived to have greater risk than a 79-year-old patient[28]
Specialty bias	Physicians are more likely to favor treatments within their scope of practice	Radiation oncologists favor radiation in the treatment of soft tissue sarcomas[10]

Adapted from Blumenthal-Barby JS, Krieger H. Cognitive biases and heuristics in medical decision making: a critical review using a systematic search strategy. Med Decis Making. 2015;35(4):539-557. https://doi.org/10.1177/0272989X14547740; with permission.

similar impact on surgical care.[6] Despite reports that cognitive bias contributes to a significant proportion of medical error, the impact is likely still underestimated given that some cognitive biases contribute in ways that do not result in measurable medical error. In a study presenting hypothetical clinical vignettes to orthopedic surgeons, several cognitive biases were noted including *base-rate neglect* and *confirmation bias*. *Base-rate neglect* describes the tendency to ignore how common or uncommon something is within a general population when viewing an individual case. *Confirmation bias* is the tendency to look for information that supports one's prior beliefs. In an example of *base-rate neglect*, 60% of surgeons studied overestimated the prevalence of uncommon diseases in interpreting test results.[8] *Confirmation bias* was apparent in that surgeons were more likely to perform confirmatory tests for a leading diagnosis rather than other diagnostic maneuvers that may contradict or disprove that diagnosis.[8] As a result, a patient may be labeled with one diagnosis without systematic consideration and elimination of other possibilities.

Cognitive bias has also been described in surgical decision-making after the initial diagnosis. An observational study of pediatric cardiothoracic care conferences, where cases were discussed among key team members, demonstrated *anchoring bias* in surgical planning. This bias resulted in inconsistency of decision-making for patients with identical diagnoses and variable decision-making for individually complex patients.[9] Physicians are likely to anchor on interventions within their scope of expertise. Therefore, surgeons are more likely to favor surgery or surgical diagnoses than their nonsurgical colleagues, a phenomenon described as *specialty bias*. For instance, in a survey of treatment recommendations for soft tissue sarcomas, radiation oncologists were likely to favor radiation therapy, medical oncologists were more likely to favor chemotherapy, and surgical oncologists placed the least emphasis on chemotherapy in a patient's overall treatment plan.[10] Similarly, in the treatment of prostate cancer, radiation oncologists and urologists view their respective treatment modalities (radiation vs surgery) as more effective and leading to a better quality-of-life than the alternative specialty's treatment modality across all risk groups.[11] In a study examining orthopedic injuries in the pediatric population, pediatric surgeons are more likely to favor early operative management of childhood sports-related injuries than sports medicine physicians, who favor nonoperative management.[12]

Cognitive bias resulting in surgical overtreatment may occur due to *commission bias* or the tendency toward action over inaction. This bias may lead to unnecessary surgical intervention, a phenomenon that has borne out in investigations of low-grade basal cell skin cancers. Dermatologic surgeons are more likely to favor invasive operative management of these lesions over nonsurgical options such as topical treatments, which are equivalent in terms of long-term disease outcomes.[13] Given that the persistent use of low-value care and high levels of overtreatment are significant contributors to the waste of health care dollars in the United States,[14] it is plausible that *commission bias* has implications not only on patient care outcomes but may also contribute to the financial impact of surgical care delivery in our health care system.

Once a patient and surgeon enter the postoperative phase of surgical care, cognitive bias continues to play an important role in the development and identification of postoperative complications. One study evaluating the incidence of cognitive bias resulting in surgical complications found that up to a third of surgical cases with a postoperative complication could be attributed to the introduction of cognitive bias in retrospective analysis.[15] Another study by the same authors compared the incidence of cognitive bias in severity-matched postoperative complications using Clavien–Dindo scores. When cognitive bias was identified, the severity of harm was higher.[16] Together these data suggest that not only does cognitive bias lead to post-operative complications but may also result in greater severity of those complications. This is possibly due to the frequency with which cognitive bias goes unrecognized without formal recognition and mitigation strategies in place.

Cognitive Bias Resulting in Delayed Diagnosis and Delay in Surgery

Amid the COVID-19 pandemic, a 43-year-old man without significant medical history presented with a fever, cough, hypoxic respiratory failure, and bilateral infiltrates on chest x-ray. He was admitted with presumed COVID-19 infection, despite initially negative testing. The patient was ultimately diagnosed with infectious mitral valve endocarditis with papillary muscle rupture requiring emergent mitral valve replacement.[17]

This clinical vignette is an example of *anchoring bias* or the tendency to base clinical decisions on the first piece of diagnostic information: in this case, hypoxic respiratory failure in the setting of the COVID-19 pandemic. It is also illustrative of *default bias* or the tendency to maintain the "status quo" during diagnostic workup. As was recently demonstrated in the COVID-19 pandemic, the novel and prevalent virus became the status quo of the health care system and therefore central in diagnostic evaluations. Similarly, *availability* and *recency biases* were at play in this clinical scenario, given that patients seen immediately before this one likely presented with the pandemic virus. In this case, superimposed cognitive biases resulted in the delayed recognition of an acute surgical illness, thus delaying appropriate and timely intervention. In cases like this, delayed surgical diagnosis can pose significant risk, particularly if the patient has an urgent or emergent condition.

Another case similarly describes severe aortic regurgitation misdiagnosed as pneumonia and fluid overload in a woman with chronic obstructive pulmonary disease and end-stage renal disease (ESRD), directly leading to delayed surgical intervention. Her pulmonary history led the team to anchor on a primary pulmonary process. When the treatment of pneumonia did not improve her volume status, her overload was misattributed to a malfunctioning dialysis catheter, thus delaying her cardiac diagnosis and eventual aortic valve replacement even further.[18] Here, we see the *default bias* of maintaining the status quo of the primary diagnosis of pneumonia and *anchoring* to her underlying condition of ESRD. This practice of not questioning a prior diagnosis is referred to as *diagnostic momentum* and has been reported, in cases like these, to prolong surgical delay.[15]

In another case of *diagnostic momentum*, an elderly man with several comorbidities presented with orthopnea quickly diagnosed as congestive heart failure (CHF) and was initiated on a diuretic regimen, which failed to clinically improve his presenting symptoms. The initial CHF diagnosis demonstrates *anchoring bias* in the setting of an elderly, comorbid man with orthopnea. However, when positional hypoxia was found incidentally during a sleep study, further workup revealed a patent foramen ovale (PFO). PFO closure was completed with the immediate relief of symptoms. *Anchoring bias* and *diagnostic momentum* supported an inaccurate CHF diagnosis and delayed appropriate surgical intervention.[19] In other circumstances, *diagnostic momentum* is generated by the context in which a patient presents. For instance, a 3-week-old neonate with hypertension was urgently referred to the inpatient cardiomyopathy service for "suspected cardiomyopathy" as opposed to "hypertension in a newborn," thus setting the stage for *framing bias*, as the suggested diagnosis likely influenced the initial diagnostic impression.[20] In this case, the patient had persistently elevated blood pressure and was transferred to the ICU where further workup revealed a left renal mass requiring nephrectomy, ultimately confirming a diagnosis of Wilms' tumor. A referral for persistent hypertension in a neonate (instead of "suspected cardiomyopathy") may have allowed for systematic consideration of diagnoses including Wilms' tumor and, as a result, more timely diagnosis and surgical intervention.

Confirmation bias is a related phenomenon in which expectations inform perception of reality. For example, a 90-year-old man with several neurovascular risk factors and poor medication adherence was well-known to an ED for hypertensive urgency. When he presented to the ED on one occasion with unilateral extremity numbness, computed tomography (CT) brain did not show acute changes. Anchoring bias led the team to diagnose transient ischemic attack and discontinue further diagnostic workup. The patient's neurologic symptoms returned and were eventually diagnosed as critical limb ischemia in the setting of arterial clot requiring emergent thromboembolectomy, delayed given his initial misdiagnosis.[21]

Across the range of surgical subspecialties, each of these cases demonstrates instances in which misdiagnosis secondary to cognitive error delayed surgical intervention.[22,23] As diagnosis and treatment proceed in the context of biases, surgical delays may have significant short-term and long-term consequences.

Cognitive Bias Resulting in Unnecessary Surgery

A healthy 28-year-old woman had a cesarean section and was admitted 7 days later for sepsis with a tender and discolored scar. Her wound was aggressively debrided given concern for necrotizing fasciitis despite persistently negative wound cultures. She underwent 10 separate surgical debridement procedures with worsening of her condition and complications ranging from anasarca to acute blood loss requiring transfusion of 13 units of blood. Ultimately, the wound was re-diagnosed as pyoderma gangrenosum, an inflammatory condition that requires immunosuppression and worsens dramatically with surgery. Her condition improved rapidly with appropriate steroid treatment.[24]

As was previously described as specialty bias, surgical diagnosis begets surgical intervention. In other words, error in surgical diagnosis may lead to an operation that is not indicated. As any surgeon well knows, surgical interventions are not without risk; thus, cognitive bias resulting in an unnecessary operation may also lead to associated downstream complications. In the above vignette, a truncated history led to an incorrect diagnosis complicated by nearly a dozen unnecessary debridement procedures, several postoperative complications, and a delay in appropriate treatment. This story also contains instances of anchoring and availability biases. In the case, the team anchored to the combination of sepsis plus wound tenderness and discoloration. Clinicians on the team also relied on the available diagnoses in their diagnostic process and obviously, could not diagnose a condition they had not considered. Moreover, clinicians are routinely less likely to consider infrequently encountered diagnoses (ie, surgical teams diagnose necrotizing fasciitis much more frequently than pyoderma gangrenosum). For the former case, debridement is crucial and may be an appropriate automatic response in many instances, yet for the latter, operative intervention dramatically worsens the condition. Similarly, confirmation bias leads us to pay closer attention to data that support our beliefs than to data that contradict them. Believing that this patient's wound was an extremely aggressive case of necrotizing fasciitis made more sense to the team initially than considering a less common diagnosis. When combined, cognitive errors compound, and doubling down on an incorrect diagnosis when the patient did not improve led to further interventions that were ultimately inappropriate and caused harm.

Several similar examples of cognitive errors resulting in unnecessary surgery are reported in the literature. One such case describes the misdiagnosis of cholangitis in a 15-year-old girl.[25] The team anchored on an elevated bilirubin and a CT scan that showed gallbladder abnormalities despite a lack of evidence for gallstones on ultrasound. *Confirmation bias* in favor of cholangitis explains the disproportionate attention paid to the patient's fever, hyperbilirubinemia, and radiologic gallbladder abnormalities at the expense of other findings. The patient was ultimately diagnosed with mononucleosis complicated by hepatitis and disseminated intravascular coagulation, an uncommon but recognized complication of Epstein–Barr virus. Just as the patient with pyoderma gangrenosum was initially diagnosed with a condition more familiar to surgeons (*availability bias*), this patient was diagnosed with cholangitis in the absence of gallstones without systematic consideration of other possibilities.

In an instance of *anchoring bias*, a patient with pulmonary sarcoidosis presented with dyspnea and hemoptysis.[26] *Anchoring bias* compounded by *default bias* and *diagnostic momentum* resulted in maintenance of the pulmonary sarcoidosis diagnosis and the patient was treated with high-dose steroids. When his condition did not improve, further workup revealed atrial perforation consistent with granulomatous infiltration. Surgical repair was performed. Ultimately, pathology revealed cardiac angiosarcoma with metastases to the brain and lungs, negating the prior diagnosis of sarcoidosis and rendering the cardiac surgery, in retrospect, futile.[26]

In another presentation of dyspnea, a patient was diagnosed with community-acquired pneumonia. When antibiotics did not improve the patient's leukocytosis and fever, further workup revealed an aortic aneurysm, enlarged from prior imaging, with ascending dissection. *Primacy effect,* or the idea that our initial ideas are manipulated to remain consistent with subsequent information, explain the team's momentum toward cardiothoracic surgery despite unexplained lymphadenopathy and concerning imaging findings. After surgical repair and several postoperative complications, an invasive endobronchial mass was diagnosed as end-stage lung cancer, a diagnosis that would have precluded surgical intervention.[27] For each of these patients, cognitive biases created inertia toward surgery that was ultimately not in the patients' best interest.

Cognitive Bias in the Operating Room and Beyond: Intraoperative Error and Surgical Complications

On the other end of the care continuum, cognitive error may also stop momentum toward a needed surgical intervention. For example, *left-digit bias*, or the tendency to categorize numerical variables by their leftmost digit, may lead a surgeon to categorize a 79-year-old patient as "in their 70s" and an 80-year-old patient as "in their 80s" in preoperative risk assessment. A study on coronary artery bypass grafts (CABGs) performed on patients 2 weeks before versus 2 weeks after their 80th birthdays demonstrated that significantly fewer patients underwent CABG after their 80th birthdays. Interestingly, this difference was not observed for birthdays without a change in leftmost digit (ie, 79th birthday or 81st birthday).[28]

Surgeons are also subject to cognitive bias in the operating room itself. One such error is *visual misperception* or "seeing what you believe."[29] Perhaps the most salient example is illustrated by surgeon estimation of volumes, rendering surgeons vulnerable to inaccurate blood loss estimates.[30] Surgeons may also "see what they believe" in anatomic identification. For example, a review of laparoscopic bile duct injury indicates the most common cause of injury is duct misidentification intraoperatively.[29] Surgical decision-making is also influenced by *overconfidence bias*, the belief that one is better than average, and *optimism bias*, the expectation of a good outcome. One study demonstrates the belief that one has an anastomotic leak rate lower than average is an independent predictor of less frequent diverting stoma formation.[31,32] Although it is logical that a surgeon who expects a positive outcome and is confident in their ability may not create a diverting loop, a study of colorectal cases with anastomotic leak ironically showed that most cases had identifiable cognitive errors, including *overconfidence bias*.[33] In another study of postoperative complications after a variety of surgeries, cognitive biases were identified in 35% of cases.[34] As previously discussed, prior work in this area has demonstrated that a significant percentage of postoperative complications are attributable to the introduction of cognitive bias and postoperative complications associated with cognitive biases result in more severe patient harm.[15,16]

Cognitive bias also plays a role in our reflection on surgical events when these events are recalled or discussed after the fact. When the surgical team reflects on major events in the operating room, data indicate individuals are universally inaccurate in their recollection of major details of the case, including the presence or absence of adverse events.[35] This phenomenon is called *recall bias*, and data suggest it is universally present as early as 1 week postoperatively.[35] This has major implications on identifying cognitive biases which may have played a role in surgical complications, and particularly so for morbidity and mortality conferences that are delivered in a delayed fashion after the clinical case itself.

Cognitive Dissonance: A Related but Distinct Phenomenon

Cognitive bias may generate cognitive dissonance, which describes the tension we experience when we hold two or more conflicting beliefs at the same time.[36] Both cognitive bias and cognitive dissonance impact the ways in which we diagnose illness preoperatively, treat disease in the operating room, and later evaluate patient outcomes postoperatively. Cognitive dissonance may intersect with the *placebo effect* and *commission bias*, or the belief that action is superior to inaction. For example, if a surgeon believes an operation will benefit a patient (potential *commission bias*) and the patient experiences subjective improvement (potential placebo effect[37,38]), then cognitive dissonance may occur if evidence for the operation performed is contradictory.[39] In a commentary piece, a prominent orthopedic surgeon describes this precise phenomenon in the case of vertebroplasty for osteoporotic vertebral compression fractures. Several clinical trials have shown that vertebroplasty for this indication is no more effective than sham surgery, yet the author describes strong, consistent personal experience of dramatic symptomatic improvement for patients.[37] His conflicting beliefs in (1) evidence-based medicine as a principle and (2) his own clinical experience that the procedure offers dramatic clinical benefit together generate cognitive dissonance and he reflects on whether he should continue to perform the procedure in question.

Commission bias also intersects with cognitive dissonance in the context of clinician decision-making for critically ill patients in the intensive care unit. In the intensive care unit, bias and dissonance may lead physicians to continue to intervene in the face of objective evidence that interventions are ineffective and prognosis is poor.[40] In one case, a patient with postoperative anastomotic leak underwent abdominal washout and several repeat operations despite poor clinical prognosis, indicating the tendency toward action over inaction.[40] This phenomenon, escalation of commitment, is defined as irrational decision-making marked by the continued allocation of resources toward a futile case.[40] Deciding which interventions are futile versus potentially lifesaving is extremely challenging for teams with a desire to "hold out hope," complicating the cascade of decision-making associated with action versus inaction. Given most ICU costs are incurred during a patient's last week of life,[40] it is likely that escalation of commitment is a common phenomenon in the ICU with implications on not only cost but also quality of life for the patient and the overall end-of-life experience for caregivers and family members.

Cognitive dissonance underlies not only clinician decision-making, but also patient decision-making. One study demonstrated this phenomenon for patients with surgical diseases including carotid artery stenosis and abdominal aortic aneurysm. For these patients, cognitive dissonance arises from the conflicting ideas that first, they "feel" healthy and, second, that a concerned surgeon believes an operation is necessary. As patients think about their own health and make medical decisions for themselves, these conflicting ideas and the cognitive dissonance they produce must be negotiated into concordance. This dissonance impacts surgical decision-making in that patients must either seek more care than they believe they need or less care than their concerned physician feels they need. In other words, patients must either proceed with "how they feel" or the physician's recommendation.

Clinical Relevance and Opportunities for Improvement

Debiasing and Patient-Facing Counseling

Shared decision-making, or medical decision-making between patient and clinician based on the patient's own values and preferences, has grown in prominence as a key component of patient-centered health care. However, biases influence the ways that clinicians approach difficult conversations and may sway patient decision-making as a result. Several studies have examined the role of *framing bias* in shared decision-making, or the idea that the way in which information is presented influences a patient's ultimate decision.[41–43] For example, extremity sarcomas may be treated with amputation or limb salvage and this decision is made between patient and clinician. Results from simulated vignettes showed descriptions framed by "functional loss" versus "functional gain" significantly impacted respondents' treatment preferences.[41] A systematic review on positive versus negative framing biases in oncology patient decision-making similarly found that positive framing led patients to choose surgery, whereas negative framing led patients to choose nonsurgical therapy.[42] For robotic surgery, in particular, data demonstrate that patients prefer robot-assisted surgery when it is described with words that highlight novelty, even when no clinical advantage to its use exists.[43] In another patient population, when a kidney for transplant is labeled as "suboptimal" with a high Kidney Donor Profile Index, many experts believe the risk–benefit is worth proceeding with transplantation for certain patients. However, patients assign a disproportionately increased risk, thus leading to unnecessarily higher organ discard rates.[44]

In addition to framing bias, *availability bias* may also influence patient decision-making. When Angelina Jolie announced she planned to undergo a bilateral prophylactic mastectomy to reduce her risk of breast cancer, interest in preventive surgical intervention for elevated breast cancer risk (ie, bilateral mastectomy) drastically increased.[45] *Availability bias* and *base-rate neglect* may have played a role by altering women's perceptions of the likelihood of developing breast cancer, thus leading more women to seek out drastic preventive measures such as prophylactic surgery.[45] Bias also influences clinicians' perceptions of prognosis. A study of oncologists demonstrated consistent *anchoring bias* during prognostication of patients with cancer, including significantly different estimates of life expectancy based on the number of months that patients stated they hoped to survive.[46] For instance, if a patient expressed desire to survive more than 30 months as opposed to 2 months, then oncologist was more likely to give a more favorable prognosis.[46] Variable numbers in prognostication are likely to have a strong effect on how patients proceed with treatment decision-making.[46]

Debiasing of the *framing effect* has been studied explicitly to neutralize unintentional clinician influence on patient decision-making. A systematic review showed that a "justification intervention" requiring patients to write a pro and con list of their options eliminated clinician *framing effect*.[42] Another study prompted clinicians to give treatment information using both positive and negative frames simultaneously, which the study team called "mixed framing." In all studies described by the review, mixed framing did not eliminate the *framing effect*. Instead, mixed framing resulted in the same decision outcome as was made with positive framing and a significantly different decision than when coached with negative framing.[42]

Other Debiasing Strategies and Surgical Practice

As described previously, cognitive processes may be broken into two categories: "system one" or "fast" thinking and "system two" or "slow" thinking.[1] Cognitive biases arise from an overreliance on system one thinking; we use the "fast" part of our brain that is programmed to jump to a conclusion quickly using recognizable patterns at the expense of our analytical "slow" brain that thinks critically. Fast thinking in surgery is often necessary, but as we have explored through the examples above, may lead to critical errors in patient care across the entire surgical spectrum.

Given the high-stakes nature of surgical decision-making and potential consequences of impaired reasoning, there is a clear need to implement effective debiasing strategies. One evidence-based strategy is to practice "meta-cognition," or thinking about how we think to recognize the influence of cognitive biases.[47] The goal of this strategy is to shift fast, system one thinking into analytical, system two thinking. Forcing decision-makers to slow down has shown encouraging results in a variety of studies, including studies on diagnostic accuracy.[5] Metacognition asks individuals to quite literally pause and "think twice" before making a decision.

Perhaps the widest implementation of a "pause" to deliberately slow thinking is the use of checklists (often termed "time-outs") in the perioperative space. A 19-item checklist designed to improve surgical team communication and consistency has been shown to reduce rates of death and postoperative complications across a range of surgical settings.[48] The implementation of similar checklists before procedures such as central line placement, management of patients on mechanical ventilation, and completion of daily tasks in the intensive care unit has also dramatically reduced morbidity and mortality.[49] In each of these cases, a checklist imposes a deliberate pause and transition to system two thinking during procedures well-trained surgeons may otherwise complete automatically via system one thinking.

Several additional debiasing strategies have been proposed but with less robust implementation, including systematic consideration of a differential diagnosis and algorithmic guidelines to guide decision-making.[5,50] Clinicians may ask themselves, "what else could this be?" or "how confident am I on a scale of one to 10?" The evidence supports the idea that deliberately interrogating one's own decision-making increases accuracy and reduces bias.[5] Formal education in biases and statistics has also been proposed as a debiasing strategy,[5] yet interventions based on increasing understanding and awareness of specific biases failed to show improved decision-making through reduction of those biases.[5] Instead, debiasing requires real-time, active effort on the part of the decision-maker.

Future Directions

As our world becomes more automated through the use of digital technology, decision support tools such as checklists and diagnostic algorithms are increasingly embedded in the electronic health record (EHR). Clinical informatics is a growing field of information technology leveraged by clinicians to deliver health care services.[51] The role of informatics in surgery, specifically, is also rapidly expanding. Already, artificial intelligence (AI) influences surgical decision-making through EHR medication dosing suggestions, drug–drug interaction alerts, and computerized outputs such as real-time vital sign graphing and postoperative anticoagulation recommendations. As the field of surgical informatics grows, some experts expect AI to become an increasingly important tool in clinical decision support. For instance, AI may increase the use of clinical support tools which would otherwise require time-intensive data entry. Such technology may be applicable to preoperative risk assessment, operative planning, and postoperative management.[52,53]

AI has the potential to reduce the margin of human error. As described in our discussion of intraoperative error, surgeons are frequently inaccurate in the recollection of major case details just 1 week postoperatively, demonstrating *recall bias*.[35] AI is already being used intraoperatively in some neurosurgical settings to augment clinician workflow and boost surgical performance.[54] For example, an optical imaging workflow has been developed that predicts intraoperative tissue biopsy diagnosis in less than 3 minutes with an overall accuracy comparable to conventional histology workflow.[55] AI has also been suggested to have a role in intraoperative charting to increase reliability in documentation of case details.[22,23] Similarly, data suggest surgeons are inaccurate in estimating volumes and surface areas intraoperatively.[30] Surgeon informaticians are actively researching the use of machine learning algorithms to reliably estimate colonic polyp size on endoscopic images. If this system proves to be reliable and reproducible, AI could improve surgeon estimation of size and volume thus reducing well-established *visual misperception bias*.[56]

Despite these promising applications, the impact of AI on cognitive biases is difficult to predict. Although automation may reduce some kinds of human error, cognitive biases are based on heuristics developed from the same pattern recognition processes implicit in machine learning.[52] As a result, AI may be subject to the same cognitive biases troubling humans.[57] In a study of the patient perspective, diagnostic accuracy was ironically perceived by patients to be both the greatest strength and the greatest weakness of AI,[58] reflecting a simultaneous trust and distrust of human cognitive ability. Interestingly, 94% of those included in the study expressed a desire for AI in medicine to be used not in isolation, but rather in conjunction with human input.[58] Thus, it seems that clinical informatics and AI are not a definitive response to cognitive biases in surgery but may serve as a promising adjunct when used in the appropriate clinical setting. However, we must also remain vigilant in slowing down, raising questions, and thinking about how we think.

CLINICS CARE POINTS

- Practicing "meta-cognition," or thinking about how we think, has been shown to reduce cognitive bias in surgery and improve diagnostic accuracy. The goal of this strategy is to slow down and "think twice" before making a clinical decision.

- Using checklists consistently in a variety of settings encourages methodical thinking and improves outcomes when used prior to procedures and operations or for daily intensive care unit tasks.

- Ask oneself "what else could this be?" or "how confident am I on a scale of 1 to 10?" when making diagnoses or clinical decisions.

- Encouraging patients to write a pro and con list of their surgical options has been shown to reduce unintentional clinician influence on decision-making.

DISCLOSURE

The authors have nothing to disclose.

REFERENCES

1. Kahneman D. Thinking, fast and slow. 1st edition. New York City, NY: Farrar, Straus and Giroux; 2011.
2. Evans JSBT. In two minds: dual-process accounts of reasoning. Trends Cogn Sci 2003;7(10):454–9.
3. Hughes TM, Dossett LA, Hawley ST, et al. Recognizing Heuristics and Bias in Clinical Decision-making. Ann Surg 2020;271(5):813–4.
4. Pitlick M, Stephenson C. 2301 Hepatic Adenoma Misdiagnosed as Biliary Colic. Off J Am Coll Gastroenterol ACG 2019;114:S1285.
5. O'Sullivan ED, Schofield SJ. Cognitive bias in clinical medicine. J R Coll Physicians Edinb 2018;48(3):225–32.
6. Graber ML, Franklin N, Gordon R. Diagnostic error in internal medicine. Arch Intern Med 2005;165(13):1493–9.
7. Blumenthal-Barby JS, Krieger H. Cognitive biases and heuristics in medical decision making: a critical review using a systematic search strategy. Med Decis Mak Int J Soc Med Decis Mak 2015;35(4):539–57.
8. Janssen SJ, Teunis T, Ring D, et al. Cognitive Biases in Orthopaedic Surgery. J Am Acad Orthop Surg 2021;29(14):624–33.
9. Duignan S, Ryan A, O'Keeffe D, et al. Prospective analysis of decision making during joint cardiology cardiothoracic conference in treatment of 107 consecutive children with congenital heart disease. Pediatr Cardiol 2018;39(7):1330–8.
10. Wasif N, Smith CA, Tamurian RM, et al. Influence of physician specialty on treatment recommendations in the multidisciplinary management of soft tissue sarcoma of the extremities. JAMA Surg 2013;148(7):632–9.
11. Kim SP, Gross CP, Nguyen PL, et al. Specialty bias in treatment recommendations and quality of life among radiation oncologists and urologists for localized prostate cancer. Prostate Cancer Prostatic Dis 2014;17(2):163–9.
12. Stinson ZS, Davelaar CMF, Kiebzak GM, et al. treatment decisions in pediatric sports medicine: do personal and professional bias affect decision-making? Orthop J Sports Med 2021;9(10). 23259671211046256.
13. Butt S, Affleck A. Decision-making in dermatologic surgery. Australas J Dermatol 2021;62(4):e568–71.
14. Shrank WH, Rogstad TL, Parekh N. Waste in the US Health Care System: Estimated Costs and Potential for Savings. JAMA 2019;322(15):1501–9.
15. Antonacci AC, Dechario SP, Antonacci C, et al. Cognitive Bias Impact on Management of Postoperative Complications, Medical Error, and Standard of Care. J Surg Res 2021;258:47–53.
16. Antonacci AC, Dechario SP, Rindskopf D, et al. Cognitive bias and severity of harm following surgery: Plan for workflow debiasing strategy. Am J Surg 2021; 222(6):1172–7.
17. Medamana JL, Leone S, Vani A, et al. A farewell to ards: papillary muscle rupture from infective endocarditis masquerading as covid pneumonia. J Am Coll Cardiol 2021;77(18):1985.
18. Narayan A, Tejani M. Shortness of breath-a critical cause obfuscated by comorbidities. J Hosp Med 2018;13(4). Available at: https://www.embase.com/search/results?subaction=viewrecord&id=L629665512&from=export.

19. Hasan R, Vallurupalli S. A year of sleeping in the recliner: Not another case of heart failure. J Am Coll Cardiol 2018;71(11). https://doi.org/10.1016/S0735-1097(18)33067-5.

20. Al Balushi A, Cunningham C, Gowrishankar M, et al. Hypertension masquerading as Pediatric Cardiomyopathy: an exercise in cognitive biases. Cardiol Young 2021;31(6):1036–8.

21. Ukaigwe A, Espana-Schmidt C. Anchoring heuristics in diagnosis. J Gen Intern Med 2014;29:S317 ((Ukaigwe A.; Espana-schmidt C.) reading health system, West Reading, PA, United States).

22. Balakrishnan K, Arjmand EM. The impact of cognitive and implicit bias on patient safety and quality. Otolaryngol Clin North Am 2019;52(1):35–46.

23. Kinaga J. Just another case of endocarditis. J Am Coll Cardiol 2019;73(9 Supplement 1):2893.

24. Berryman J, Hilton R, Handoyo K. Pyoderma gangrenosum mimicking necrotizing fasciitis: A case of anchoring bias. J Gen Intern Med 2017;32(2):S574.

25. Graber ML, Berg D, Jerde W, et al. Learning from tragedy: the Julia Berg story. Diagn Berl Ger 2018;5(4):257–66.

26. Sutter J, Rao A, Clark B. A confounding diagnosis: cardiac angiosarcoma mistaken for sarcoidosis. J Am Coll Cardiol 2020;75(11):3412.

27. Riggs J, Steiner S, Oppenheimer B. Anchoring to death: An unfortunate case of predecisional information distortion in the diagnosis of end-stage lung cancer. Am J Respir Crit Care Med 2017;195. https://doi.org/10.1164/ajrccmconference.2017.C57. Riggs J., jarigg@gmail.com; Steiner S.) NYU Langone Medical Center, New York, NY, United States.

28. Olenski AR, Zimerman A, Coussens S, et al. Behavioral heuristics in coronary-artery bypass graft surgery. N Engl J Med 2020;382(8):778–9.

29. Dekker SWA, Hugh TB. Laparoscopic bile duct injury: understanding the psychology and heuristics of the error. ANZ J Surg 2008;78(12):1109–14.

30. Schuld J, Kollmar O, Seidel R, et al. Estimate or calculate? How surgeons rate volumes and surfaces. Langenbecks Arch Surg 2012;397(5):763–9.

31. MacDermid E, Young CJ, Moug SJ, et al. Heuristics and bias in rectal surgery. Int J Colorectal Dis 2017;32(8):1109–15.

32. MacDermid E, Young CJ, Young J, et al. Decision-making in rectal surgery. Colorectal Dis Off J Assoc Coloproctol G B Irel 2014;16(3):203–8.

33. Vogel P, Vogel DHV. Cognition errors in the treatment course of patients with anastomotic failure after colorectal resection. Patient Saf Surg 2019;13:4.

34. Siskind S, Thompson D, Bolourani S, et al. Cognitive Bias in Management of Cases Sustaining Postoperative Complication. J Am Coll Surg 2020;231(4):S242.

35. Alsubaie H, Goldenberg M, Grantcharov T. Quantifying recall bias in surgical safety: a need for a modern approach to morbidity and mortality reviews. Can J Surg J Can Chir 2019;62(1):39–43.

36. Byrne PJ. The Role of Objective Outcomes in Surgery in Overcoming Cognitive Dissonance. JAMA Facial Plast Surg 2016;18(3):163–4.

37. Orr RD. Vertebroplasty, cognitive dissonance, and evidence-based medicine: what do we do when the "evidence" says we are wrong? Cleve Clin J Med 2010;77(1):8–11.

38. Moseley JB, O'Malley K, Petersen NJ, et al. A Controlled Trial of Arthroscopic Surgery for Osteoarthritis of the Knee. N Engl J Med 2002;347(2):81–8.

39. Homer JJ, Sheard CE, Jones NS. Cognitive dissonance, the placebo effect and the evaluation of surgical results. Clin Otolaryngol Allied Sci 2000;25(3):195–9.

40. Braxton CC, Robinson CN, Awad SS. Escalation of Commitment in the Surgical ICU. Crit Care Med 2017;45(4):e433–6.
41. Gurich RW, Cizik AM, Punt SE, et al. Decision-making in orthopaedic oncology: does cognitive bias affect a virtual patient's choice between limb salvage and amputation? Clin Orthop 2020;478(3):506–14.
42. Tang YT, Chooi WT. A systematic review of the effects of positive versus negative framing on cancer treatment decision making. Psychol Health 2021;1–26. https://doi.org/10.1080/08870446.2021.2006197. Tang Y.-T.; Chooi W.-T. School of Social Sciences, Universiti Sains Malaysia, Pulau Pinang, Malaysia.
43. Dixon PR, Grant RC, Urbach DR. The impact of marketing language on patient preference for robot-assisted surgery. Surg Innov 2015;22(1):15–9.
44. Heilman RL, Green EP, Reddy KS, et al. Potential Impact of Risk and Loss Aversion on the Process of Accepting Kidneys for Transplantation. Transplantation 2017;101(7):1514–7.
45. Pravettoni G, Gorini A, Bonanni B, et al. The role of heuristics and biases in cancer-related decisions. Ecancermedicalscience 2013;7:ed26.
46. Shalowitz DI, Schorge JO. Suggestibility of oncologists' clinical estimates. JAMA Oncol 2015;1(2):251–3.
47. Croskerry P. From mindless to mindful practice — cognitive bias and clinical decision making. N Engl J Med 2013;368(26):2445–8.
48. Haynes AB, Weiser TG, Berry WR, et al. A surgical safety checklist to reduce morbidity and mortality in a global population. N Engl J Med 2009;360(5):491–9.
49. Gawande A. The Checklist. New Yorker 2007;83(39):86–95.
50. Croskerry P. The importance of cognitive errors in diagnosis and strategies to minimize them. Acad Med 2003;78(8):775–80.
51. Zhao J, Forsythe R, Langerman A, et al. The Value of the Surgeon Informatician. J Surg Res 2020;252:264–71.
52. Loftus TJ, Tighe PJ, Filiberto AC, et al. Artificial Intelligence and Surgical Decision-making. JAMA Surg 2020;155(2):148–58.
53. Corey KM, Kashyap S, Lorenzi E, et al. Development and validation of machine learning models to identify high-risk surgical patients using automatically curated electronic health record data (Pythia): A retrospective, single-site study. Plos Med 2018;15(11):e1002701.
54. Tariciotti L, Palmisciano P, Giordano M, et al. Artificial intelligence-enhanced intraoperative neurosurgical workflow: state of the art and future perspectives. J Neurosurg Sci 2021. https://doi.org/10.23736/S0390-5616.21.05483-7.
55. Mofatteh M. Neurosurgery and artificial intelligence. AIMS Neurosci 2021;8(4):477–95.
56. Suykens J, Eelbode T, Daenen J, et al. AUTOMATED POLYP SIZE ESTIMATION WITH DEEP LEARNING REDUCES INTEROBSERVER VARIABILITY. Gastrointest Endosc 2020;91(6):AB241–2.
57. Pérez MJ, Grande RG. Application of artificial intelligence in the diagnosis and treatment of hepatocellular carcinoma: A review. World J Gastroenterol 2020;26(37):5617–28.
58. Nelson CA, Pérez-Chada LM, Creadore A, et al. Patient Perspectives on the Use of Artificial Intelligence for Skin Cancer Screening: A Qualitative Study. JAMA Dermatol 2020;156(5):501–12.

Generation Learning Differences in Surgery
Why They Exist, Implication, and Future Directions

Mike Weykamp, MD[a], Jason Bingham, MD[b],*

KEYWORDS

- Generational learning • Learning theory • Connectivism • Artificial intelligence
- Machine learning • Asynchronous learning • Medical education
- Learning disparities

KEY POINTS

- The rapid expansion of clinical knowledge and correspondingly shortening half-life of this information is not sustainable within the traditional framework of surgical education.
- Entry and credentialing examinations create pressures on learners to seek proven, efficient learning materials, often at expense of in-person, program-sponsored curricula; the contents, format, and utility of these examinations deserve scrutiny.
- Professionally produced and vetted digital/audiovisual medical education content has the potential to improve learner efficiency, offload clinical instructors, and address disparities in access to high-quality instruction.
- Artificial intelligence, machine learning, and computerized decision support tools will play an increased role in surgical training and practice in the future, thoughtful evaluation and implementation of these technologies should be embraced by the surgical community.

INTRODUCTION

In the little more than 150 years since safe anesthesia and antisepsis practices made the modern practice of surgery possible, there has been an exponential increase in surgical knowledge. This expansion in knowledge, in combination with technological advances, and the evolution of medical accreditation and licensing processes, among other factors, have driven change in the methods by which surgeons are educated. The speed of this change has been such that the learning environment occupied by

[a] Department of Surgery, University of Washington, 1959 NE Pacific Street, Seattle, WA 98195, USA; [b] Uniformed Services University of Health Sciences, 4301 Jones Bridge Road, Bethesda, MD 20814, USA
* Corresponding author. Department of General Surgery, Madigan Army Medical Center, 9040 Jackson Avenue, Tacoma, WA 98431.
E-mail address: jrpbingham@gmail.com

Surg Clin N Am 103 (2023) 287–298
https://doi.org/10.1016/j.suc.2022.11.008
0039-6109/23/Published by Elsevier Inc.

contemporary surgical learners is often unrecognizable to even the faculty from whom they are learning.

The resulting disconnect in learning styles between generations of surgeons has important implications for the future of surgery and warrants the attention of the surgical community to ensure that the ongoing evolution of surgical education continues to produce clinicians equipped to rise the challenges of the modern surgical practice. Although the focus of this article is on how generational learning differences impact surgery specifically, as the factors that drive these differences are apparent long before one enters a surgical training program, the following exploration of this topic will include concepts from premedical education and beyond.

THE EXPONENTIAL GROWTH OF KNOWLEDGE

The sheer volume of new surgery-related knowledge is arguably the most powerful driver of change in surgical education. Since shortly after the end of World War II, there has been an explosion of surgical literature informing the state of the art which trainees must master (**Fig. 1**).[1] The current surgical workforce straddles the inflection point of this exponential growth curve, with the average clinical professor being approximately 61 years old according to the 2022 US Medical Faculty AAMC report.[2] For the purposes of illustrating the magnitude of this generational difference, if a 61-year-old professor of surgery in 2022 graduated medical school in 1987 (at age 26) there would have been 1,032,048 *total* PubMed articles indexed to the search term "Surgery" published before their internship.[1] For a surgical intern graduating medical school in 2022, there were 313,315 similar articles published in their senior year of medical school

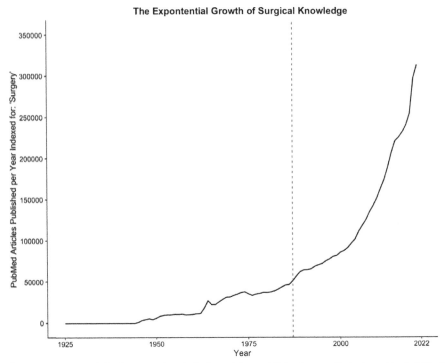

Fig. 1. Depiction of the increase in scholarly articles published annually indexed in PubMed (MEDLINE) to the search term "Surgery" over time.[1] Dashed red line (1987) approximates the medical school graduation year of current clinical professors.

alone, not to mention the 4,298,723 published in the intervening years as their professor entered the field.[1]

This acceleration in the pace of knowledge generation is associated with a corresponding decrease in the half-life of that knowledge (ie, the duration of time that an article or guideline remains current before it is replaced with more up-to-date content). Research exploring the concept of medical information obsolescence has quantified the median "survival" of guidelines and systematic reviews before new information mandates their being updated or replaced at approximately 5.5 years, with experts in medical cognitive computing predicting that the concept of medical information half-life will soon be measured in months.[3–5] This combination of knowledge expansion and decay creates obvious challenges for learners, particularly those in the early phases of their training or true generalists who must remain current in various domains of surgery. Although continuing medical education initiatives offer a partial solution to this issue, there remains an unmet need for a comprehensive information management system in surgery and the current deluge of information overwhelms the capacity of many practitioners to keep pace. This increasingly poses a threat to patient safety via the potential for the inadvertent delivery of outdated and therefore substandard care.

Although the rapid increase in primary literature production has been associated with breakthroughs in patient care and assuaged human suffering in ways that would have been unimaginable to surgical pioneers like Lister and Halsted, the motivations for producing such work have expanded to include accumulation of academic currency to be exchanged for prestige, promotion, and tenure.[6] This, among other motivations, has driven demand for outlets to publish in and a corresponding increase in the number of scholarly journals has occurred. In 2021, there were 492 surgical journals cataloged by the SCImago group's Scopus-based library up from 304 in 1999 representing more than a 60% increase in just over twenty years.[7] Although some of these publications were born out of the trend toward surgical subspecialization which we will discuss in upcoming sections, the commoditization of research productivity and the increase in publication venues has diluted the quality of the literature and increased the difficulty in identifying relevant work among the noise for modern learners compared with their predecessors.

LEARNING THEORIES

The way people acquire knowledge varies between individuals, changes over time, and is the subject of a whole field of scholarship with competing theories as to how we encode information and incorporate it into our decisions and how best to optimize these processes. Traditional learning theories include:

- Behaviorism: defines learning as "observable increases, decreases, or maintenance of behaviors" and posits that learning is largely a consequence of conditioning via an individual's interactions with their environment.[8]
- Cognitivism: defines learning as an "internal mental process" through which individuals create mental representations (schema) of their experiences that can be drawn upon in the future.[8]
- Constructivism: defines learning as the active, intentional construction of mental schema by which learners take in new information and either assimilate it within an existing schema or accommodate/create new schema based on new data, as contrasted to the more passive processes proposed by cognitivists.[8,9]

In his seminal work *Connectivism: A Learning Theory for the Digital Age*, George Siemens proposed "Connectivism" as a discrete learning theory. This represented a paradigm shift suggesting that people can learn (ie, acquire actionable information) via networks of information containing nodes that include people, technologies, or organizations rather than exclusively via one's own experiences.[10] The concept of "connectivism" arose from the idea that the knowledge on which our actions are based is constantly shifting beneath our feet and that the ability to rapidly access, triage, and incorporate knowledge from networks is at the heart of contemporary learning.[8,10]

Some observers contend that there are stylistic differences that are intrinsic to different generations of learners (**Table 1**). Specifically, the role of generational differences in adaptation to and adoption of technology is frequently commented on and is increasingly the subject of academic research.[11,12] In 2001, education and technology writer Marc Prensky coined the often-cited terminology "*digital natives*" and "*digital immigrants*" to describe those who were raised in the post-Internet, digital era, and those whose development pre-dated it (before approximately 1980), respectively.[13] Commentators of various backgrounds have endorsed the seemingly intuitive hypothesis that *digital natives* will be adept at assimilating to technological advances into their learning and work whereas the older *digital immigrants* will tend to struggle by comparison.[14] When tested scientifically in pragmatic contexts, however, the results of these studies have failed to consistently support this theory and show that so-called *digital natives* have heterogeneous learning preferences and much of their interaction with technology is superficial (eg, e-mailing, word processing, and gaming) rather than foundational to who they are as learners.[14] Interestingly, studies have also shown that so-called *digital immigrants* are able to achieve similar self-efficacy metrics with respect to the utilization of educational technologies suggesting that reservations about their capacity to participate in increasingly digital classrooms, workplaces, and society are likely overstated.[11,15,16]

THE KNOWLEDGE ECONOMY

Medical education market growth. Historically, the intergenerational transfer of medical and surgical knowledge has occurred person-to-person and face to face whether it was through formal apprenticeships, tutors for medical school quizzes in the early twentieth century, or the lectures given by expert faculty.[17] The effectiveness of these methods is contingent on both the knowledge and teaching abilities of an instructor, and the variable quality of this education style and the graduates it produced prompted the trend toward standardization of medical education via program accreditation and individual licensing at the turn of the twentieth century.[17] Although this regulation measurably improved the quality of medical and surgical care in the United States, the publication

Table 1 Learning styles by generation	
Generation (Birth Years)[a]	**Generalized Learning and Working Preferences**
Silent (1925–1942)	Structured classroom work, "top down" instruction, and disciplined[41]
Baby Boomer (1943–1960)	Incentive based tasks, independence, competition[41,42]
Generation X (1961–1981)	Efficient, flexible, clear expectations, and ability to question relevance[41,42]
Millennials (1982–1996)	Relaxed, collaborative, context provided, and multiple learning modalities[41,43–45]

Description of generalized learning styles between four generations comprising the current surgical workforce

[a] Birth year ranges are approximations; no agreed-upon birth year cutoffs defining each generation exist.

of standards and curricula effectively created a template for training physicians and in combination with the increasing competitiveness of training positions in recent years has created an environment ripe for commercialization of medical education.[18,19]

In 2020, the global medical education market was valued at USD 74.5 billion with forecasted growth to $122.8 billion in revenue by 2027 with North America making up the largest regional market share.[20] This quantifiably high and increasing demand for quality medical education content has been driven in large part by increasing competitiveness for seats in various training programs from medical school to fellowship. The commercial resources created by industry are increasingly tailored to the specifications of their end-users (efficient, high yield for entry/licensing examinations, and multimedia supported) in a way that makes it difficult for traditional faculty educators, who have competing clinical responsibilities, to rival when competing for the time and attention of trainees. Although outsourcing learning topics as critical as pathology, physiology, and anatomy to industry-generated materials is a foreign (and for some, concerning) concept to surgeons whose training occurred before the turn of the century, these materials are increasingly relied upon by contemporary learners who value their efficiency, portability, and proven track record for examination preparation.[21]

Sub-specialization. A natural consequence of the growth in surgical knowledge, the increased number of procedures offered, and their complexity has been a paradigm shift from generalist to specialist. The surgeon who performs the full breadth of procedures his or her credentials allow is increasingly an endangered species. For example, patients referred with a rectal malignancy or evaluation for bariatric surgery that were previously common in general surgery clinics are increasingly being referred to fellowship-trained subspecialists with expertise in their increasingly nuanced fields.[22] This has fundamentally changed surgical training in ways as obvious as the development of integrated training programs (eg, vascular, cardiothoracic, and plastic surgery) to more subtle, like trainee exposure to certain specialist-owned pathologies being limited to certain several-week rotations rather than traditional longitudinal exposures over the course of their training. In short, the increasing breadth and depth of surgical expertise have resulted in fragmentation of practice which has created challenges in ensuring that trainees receive the exposure, instruction, and case numbers required to achieve competence in the various domains they are responsible for on their board examinations.[22]

This organization and specialization of surgery as a field has also given rise to new surgical professional societies. These societies range from general to subspecialized, social to rigorous, and regional to international. It is common for such societies to have committees that review the evidence in their respective fields and issue best practice recommendations, literature reviews, or clinical practice guidelines. Although such efforts are inherently evidence based, it is not uncommon for different organizations to publish best practice guidelines that are discordant from peer organizations with overlapping subject matter expertise.[23,24] Although professional organizations provide a valuable service in helping to navigate the increasingly specialized literature via expert curation, review, and interpretation of the evidence, an imperfect collaboration between such organizations contributes to the cluttered information landscape with which modern learners must contend.

Although continued subspecialization seems inevitable, it is worth mentioning that the trend from generalist training to specialist training is not a panacea to addressing the increasing complexity of modern surgical practice. First, with the increasingly narrow scopes of practice of subspecialists, surgeons require a larger referral population to support their practices. This has led to the consolidation of specialists in metropolitan demographics which creates issues with inequitable access to care in rural and other underserved populations who sometimes must travel hours at significant personal expense to receive appropriate surgical care.[25] Additionally, there is the issue of ensuring adequate training to manage time-sensitive surgical emergencies. For example, with the expansion of specialties with integrated training programs like vascular surgery, general surgery trainee experience with emergent procedures like vascular shunting/repair and fasciotomies are declining.[26] With access to specialist care varying based on the hospital system, and emergency general surgery services remaining the first or only option at some centers for these procedures, continued momentum toward specialization has the potential to create a crisis of readiness for some emergent procedures among the non-specialists expected to be facile with them.

Asynchronous learning technologies. The modalities through which surgical trainees acquire knowledge increasingly include audiovisual, interactive, or searchable content delivered through electronic media. The miniaturization of devices capable of accessing this content has made it omnipresent in the cell phones and tablets of every surgical trainee. Learners can access professionally curated procedure videos, surgery podcasts, or lectures from leaders in the field on virtually any topic in real time often with variable speed playback capabilities allowing for efficient consumption of the material that can be revisited and reviewed 24/7. These resources allow for a level of efficiency that was unheard for prior generations of surgical trainees whose training occurred before wide-scale consumer computing and the maturation of the Internet.

Although these technological advances have provided some capacity to navigate the flood of information in a way that would not be possible through the textbooks and in-person lectures of prior generations, they are not without their issues. First, the generation of digital surgical content can be performed from entities as trusted as government agencies or universities to those as unpredictable as individuals with a webcam and microphone, and the peer review process for such content is variable and sometimes non-existent. Furthermore, there is no centralized process for monitoring such content and popular sites like YouTube are filled with out-of-date or incorrect medical information and surgical videos demonstrating suboptimal or even dangerous techniques.[27-29] For example, when experts reviewed the top 10 YouTube operative videos for laparoscopic cholecystectomy, they found that only one achieved the gold standard critical view of safety and noted potentially dangerous safety violations in half of the videos.[27] Finally, a future in which education relies on technology and commercially produced (often for-profit) resources risks discrimination on socioeconomic grounds against those who lack to means to access them.

Technology has also expanded into the realm of technical skill development. For reasons including patient safety, financial pressures on operating room throughput, and medical-legal issues there has been a gradual erosion in the autonomy granted to surgical learners and corresponding concerns about the readiness of residency graduates for independent practice.[30-32] Simulation technologies are increasingly being used to address these competing priorities. Traditional simulation techniques for teaching open surgical skills have ranged from low-fidelity models made of household items approximating tissues to multi-million-dollar, computer-integrated, modular human mannequin models. Although to some extent simulation is not unique to recent generations, its ubiquity in surgical training is a relatively new phenomenon compared with the "see one, do one, teach one" education of the current cadre of senior surgery faculty. This is perhaps best illustrated by the integration of formal simulation curricula in surgery training in the form of programs like Fundamentals of Laparoscopic Surgery (FLS) and Fundamentals of Endoscopic Surgery (FES) as requirements for American Board of Surgery certification as recently as 2009 and 2014, respectively.[33,34] The advent of robotic surgery has pushed simulation to the next level with modules allowing learners to complete entire operations virtually before ever laying hands on a patient.

DISCUSSION

As we have outlined, information growth and the evolution of the knowledge economy and technology industry have fundamentally changed the learning environments occupied by contemporary surgical trainees and created pressures that will force the surgical community to consider:

- Re-structuring the traditional teacher-trainee dynamic
- Defining the appropriate role of industry in medical and surgical education and embracing partnerships when appropriate
- Continued revision of entry, in-service, and licensing examination structure and content to intentionally direct the pressures they exert on learners more productively
- Incorporating technology, artificial intelligence, and computer-assisted decision support tools into practice

The differences in learning environments occupied by current surgical trainees and those that were occupied by their senior peers have several important implications. First of these is that learners and teachers often begin their relationships with incongruous expectations of one another. Instructors whose own education involved diligent preparation for, and attendance of in-person didactic sessions often view waning in-person attendance for such material as being a function of generational laziness and even disrespect. When the trainees themselves are surveyed, however, their input paints a different picture entirely. For example, when medical students were surveyed to determine the factors underlying their decisions to either attend or not attend in-person faculty lectures, Emahiser and colleagues[35] found that the most cited reason for non-attendance among these learners was the relative inefficiency of information intake compared with recorded materials. Furthermore, rather than "lazy," those endorsing a predilection for lecture non-attendance were disproportionately students with aspirations for more competitive residency programs including surgical subspecialties.[35] With the rapid quality of commercially produced educational content combined with this mutual disillusionment with in person lecture, we suggest that the question should shift from why learners attend in-person teaching or not to focusing on (1) how we best use the time of clinical instructors and (2) are high-stakes examinations that are exerting increasing influence on trainee's educational priorities evaluating what we want them to?

Is it, for example, a wise use of a clinical instructor's time to lecture surgical trainees on the basics of diagnosis and management colorectal malignancy, a topic with innumerable resources including SCORE©, TrueLearn©, Behind the Knife©, and others that cover this topic with professionally produced and vetted video lectures, audio podcasts, and interactive questions banks? With evidence supporting the disenchantment of learners and teachers alike with traditional lecture formats, and the satisfactory performance of industry-produced content for examination preparation, we suggest that valuable in-person time might be better used to clarify questions that exist after preparation with pre-prepared materials (eg, the flipped classroom model) or focusing clinical instruction on topics that are beyond the scope of industry produced content like technical skills, and interpersonal proficiency. Although the idea of effectively outsourcing medical education to industry might raise eyebrows among the old guard of surgical education, this is already happening, and embracing these relationships would allow for in-person teaching with faculty to focus on nuanced topics and interpersonal or technical skills that are beyond the capacity of the medical education industry to emulate and therefore promote engagement and understanding across generations.

Another relevant question is how the standards for what surgical trainees should learn are set. We contend that the responsibility is increasingly, though perhaps unintentionally, being abdicated to the authors of board examinations and the commercial resources learners use to prepare for them. Although examination content setting the standard for a consistent curriculum is not inherently a negative, with such examinations (eg, MCAT, USMLE step examinations, and ABSITE) increasingly being used as standardized metrics to assist in selecting candidates for training positions rather than arbiters of a baseline level of competence, the content of these examinations includes increasing amounts of intricacies of debatable utility apart from discerning between similarly qualified applicants. Although there has been some movement toward these sorts of standardized examinations becoming pass/fail to return to their initial purpose of ensuring an acceptable standard, their role as proxies for quality applicants is entrenched.[36] With the increasing breadth and depth of expertise required to be a safe surgeon in modern practice, the contents of these examinations must be carefully monitored to ensure that they are adapting to the environment in which trainees will practice with an emphasis on ensuring that time spent preparing for them is time spent developing competence rather than briefly memorizing minutiae to earn a place on the rightward tail of a bell curve. This concept has already gained momentum with the USMLE Step 1 examination, which contains large amounts of basic science or foundational science concepts moving to a pass/fail format, and the American Board of Surgery recertification examination moving to offer an online open resource option in which examinees are free to access any resource they would use in practice for the test.[36,37]

Although there is room for improvement in the way in which medical education is structured to bridge generational differences or ensure closer alignment between curricula and practice with minimal waste—the sheer speed of information growth is such that these solutions are likely only a finger in the leaky dike. Existing medical education infrastructure lacks the flexibility and resources to keep pace with the knowledge their trainees must contend with. We contend success or failure of medical education in the information age is tied to our ability to harness the only tool at our disposal to progress at a rate commensurate with information growth: processing power.

Moore's law refers to an observation credited to Gordon Moore, an Intel co-founder, in 1971 in which he forecast that the number of components per integrated circuit (a proxy for processing power) would double every two years. In the decades that followed, Moore's prediction largely proved correct (**Fig. 2**) and was associated with the birth of commercial computing and the subsequent miniaturization of computers for an array of practical applications.[38] Although these advances are apparent in surgery in the form of videoendoscopic and robotic capabilities, the application of computational advances with respect to information management (eg, artificial intelligence, machine learning, and computer-assisted decision support tools) are just scratching the surface. Although in its infancy, integration of artificial intelligence into clinical life has already begun. Computer-based decision support in the form of automated real-time electrocardiogram interpretation, electronic medical record-based drug-drug interaction alerts, and indication-based radiology order support are already commonplace in clinical practice.[39] More ambitious clinical artificial intelligence tools are actively being developed with technology companies like IBM Watson Health (New York, NY), DeepMind (London, UK), and Google (Mountain View, CA) attempting to tackle cross-sectional imaging interpretation or even comprehensive clinical decision support.[39] Early attempts at implementation of these technologies have met some resistance from physician groups, many of whom view reliance on technology in patient care as a slippery slope and cite concerns about physician skill atrophy, issues with patient safety/liability, and encroachment on their scope of

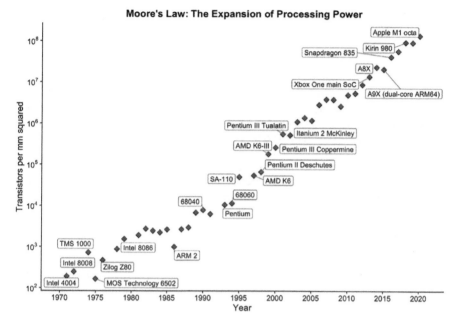

Fig. 2. Scatter plot showing the increase in transistor density over time between 1971 and 2021. Each point represents the processor with the highest transistor density released each year. Data are a subset of those presented by Eric Martin in *Moore's Law is Alive and Well*. (*Data from Martin E. Moore's Law is Alive and Well. Medium. Accessed July 26, 2022*. https://medium.com/predict/moores-law-is-alive-and-well-eaa49a450188.)

practice.[39,40] Although these concerns have merit and should be duly considered in the design and integration of any new technology into surgical practice, we suggest that the reticence to accept the increasing role of technology in the practice of medicine is in part related to the generational differences we have outlined above. Surgery has a rich tradition of skepticism and tendency to allow inertia to maintain the status quo until overwhelming evidence prompts change in practice. When based on rigorous application of the scientific method, this tendency has been largely adaptative and has prevented many unsubstantiated medications, procedures, and treatment strategies from harming patients. Although it is critically important that this due diligence be applied to the integration artificial intelligence into surgical practice, it is equally important that these solutions not be dismissed out of hand by those whose training and early practice pre-date the pressures that make them necessary reaching a critical mass.

The above discussion of learning styles, knowledge expansion, the medical information economy, and the transition into the technology-driven area of connectivism raises the critical question: what is the role of the surgical educator in this new environment? With the information required to safely practice surgery increasingly available via networks of digital content, organizational knowledge, and readily accessible clinical care guidelines the surgical educator's role will increasingly be teaching learners to effectively connect with and navigate these networks rather than serving as direct conduits of information themselves. Although the role of clinical surgical educators as stewards of technical skill and clinical decision-making will persist into the future, ensuring that their trainees are facile in navigating complex networks of ever-updating clinical evidence and capable of thoughtful incorporation of these networks in their decision-making will be as important as ensuring their competence with exposure, suturing, and tissue handling.

SUMMARY

Although there are perhaps some learning differences that are intrinsic to the generations themselves, we suggest that these differences are primarily a function of the environments in which surgeons of different generations trained. If unaddressed, the pressures driving these differences have the potential to undermine instructor-trainee relationships, existing training curricula, and the readiness of the future surgical workforce. Although the solutions to these issues must be as multifaceted as the causes, we submit that acknowledgment of the principles of connectivism and thoughtful integration of artificial intelligence and computerized decision support tools must play a central role in charting the future course of surgical education to ensure a smooth passing of the baton between generations of surgeons.

DISCLOSURE

The authors have nothing to disclose. The viewpoints expressed are those of the authors along, and do not represent the viewpoints of the University of Washington, the Uniformed Services University of Health Sciences, or the Department of Defense.

REFERENCES

1. PubMed (MEDLINE). Available at: https://pubmed-ncbi-nlm-nih-gov.offcampus.lib.washington.edu/?myncbishare=uwonline. Accessed June 1, 2022.
2. AAMC Faculty Roster. Supplemental Table H: Average Age of Full-time Faculty and Chairs by Gender, Rank, and Department Type, 2021. Association of American Medical Colleges. Available at: https://www.aamc.org/media/58541/download?attachment. Accessed 24 July 2022.
3. Shojania KG, Sampson M, Ansari MT, Ji J, Doucette S, Moher D. How quickly do systematic reviews go out of date? A survival analysis. Ann Intern Med 2007; 147(4):224–33.
4. Shekelle PG, Ortiz E, Rhodes S, et al. Validity of the Agency for Healthcare Research and Quality clinical practice guidelines: how quickly do guidelines become outdated? JAMA 2001;286(12):1461–7.
5. Sepulveda MH. Cognitive Technologies, Thinking, and Time. Harvard Medical School; 2016. Available at: https://www.youtube.com/watch?v=oPvtypHTXew. Accessed June 1, 2022.
6. Siegel MG, Brand JC, Rossi MJ, Lubowitz JH. "Publish or perish" promotes medical literature quantity over quality. Arthroscopy 2018;34(11):2941–2.
7. SCImago. SJR — SCImago Journal and Country Rank [Portal]. Available at: https://www.scimagojr.com. Accessed July 24, 2022.
8. Kay D, Kibble J. Learning theories 101: application to everyday teaching and scholarship. Advances in physiology education 2016;40(1):17–25.
9. Bada SO. Constructivism learning theory: a paradigm for teaching and learning. Journal of Research & Method in Education 2015;5(6):66–70.
10. Siemens G. Connectivism: a learning theory for the digital age. International Journal of Instructional Technology and Distance Learning [Online]. 2004. Available at: https://www.itdl.org/Journal/Jan_05/article01.htm. Accessed June 1, 2022.
11. Salajan F, Schonwetter D, Cleghorn B. Student and faculty inter-generational digital divide: Fact or fiction? Computers & Education 2010;55(3):1393–403.

12. Myers C, Conner M. Age differences in skill acquisition and transfer in an implicit learning paradigm. Applied Cognitive Psychology 1992;6(5):429–42.
13. Prensky M. Digital natives, digital immigrants part 1. On the Horizon 2001; 9(5):1–6.
14. Bennett S, Maton K, Kervin L. The 'digital natives' debate: a critical review of the evidence. British Journal of Educational Technology 2008;39(5):775–86.
15. Waycott J, Bennett S, Kennedy G, Dalgarno B, Gray K. Digital divides? Student and staff perceptions of information and communication technologies. Computers and education 2010;54(4):1202–11.
16. Guo RX, Dobson T, Petrina S. Digital natives, digital immigrants: an analysis of age and ict competency in teacher education. Journal of educational computing research 2008;38(3):235–54.
17. Camison L, Brooker J, Naran S, Potts J III, Losee J. The history of surgical education in the United States: past, present, and future. Annals of Surgery Open 2022;3(1):e148.
18. Roberts JS, Coale JG, Redman RR. A history of the joint commission on accreditation of hospitals. JAMA 1987;258(7):936–40.
19. Hussein M, Pavlova M, Ghalwash M, Groot W. The impact of hospital accreditation on the quality of healthcare: a systematic literature review. BMC Health Serv Res. Oct 6 2021;21(1):1057.
20. QYResearch. Global Medical Education Market Size, Status and Forecast 2021-2027. 2021. Available at: https://reports.valuates.com/reports/QYRE-Othe-2D465/global-medical-education. Accessed 16 July 2022.
21. Hirumi A, Horger L, Harris DM, et al. Exploring students' [pre-pandemic] use and the impact of commercial-off-the-shelf learning platforms on students' national licensing exam performance: a focused review - BEME Guide No. 72. Med Teach 2022;44(7):707–19.
22. Bruns SD, Davis BR, Demirjian AN, et al. The subspecialization of surgery: a paradigm shift. J Gastrointest Surg 2014;18(8):1523–31.
23. Galetin T, Galetin A, Vestweber KH, Rink AD. Systematic review and comparison of national and international guidelines on diverticular disease. Int J Colorectal Dis 2018;33(3):261–72.
24. Adam MA, Goffredo P, Youngwirth L, Scheri RP, Roman SA, Sosa JA. Same thyroid cancer, different national practice guidelines: When discordant American Thyroid Association and National Comprehensive Cancer Network surgery recommendations are associated with compromised patient outcome. Surgery 2016;159(1):41–50.
25. Baldwin LM, Cai Y, Larson EH, et al. Access to cancer services for rural colorectal cancer patients. J Rural Health Fall 2008;24(4):390–9.
26. Yan H, Maximus S, Koopmann M, et al. Vascular Trauma Operative Experience is Inadequate in General Surgery Programs. Ann Vasc Surg 2016;33:94–7.
27. Rodriguez HA, Young MT, Jackson HT, Oelschlager BK, Wright AS. Viewer discretion advised: is YouTube a friend or foe in surgical education? Surg Endosc 2018;32(4):1724–8.
28. Huynh D, Fadaee N, Gök H, Wright A, Towfigh S. Thou shalt not trust online videos for inguinal hernia repair techniques. Surg Endosc 2021;35(10):5724–8.
29. Jackson HT, Hung CS, Potarazu D, et al. Attending guidance advised: educational quality of surgical videos on YouTube. Surg Endosc 2022;36(6):4189–98.
30. Kempenich JW, Dent DL. General surgery resident autonomy: truth and myth. Surg Clin North Am 2021;101(4):597–609.

31. Mattar SG, Alseidi AA, Jones DB, et al. General surgery residency inadequately prepares trainees for fellowship: results of a survey of fellowship program directors. Ann Surg 2013;258(3):440–9.

32. Napolitano LM, Savarise M, Paramo JC, et al. Are general surgery residents ready to practice? A survey of the American College of Surgeons Board of Governors and Young Fellows Association. J Am Coll Surg 2014;218(5):1063–72.e31.

33. Shiffer C. ABS to Require ACLS, ATLS and FLS for General Surgery Certification. The American Board of Surgery. Available at: https://www.absurgery.org/default.jsp?news_newreqs. Accessed June 1, 2022.

34. New requirement in flexible endoscopy. The American Board of Surgery. Available at: https://www.absurgery.org/default.jsp?certgsqe_fec. Accessed June 1, 2022.

35. Emahiser J, Nguyen J, Vanier C, Sadik A. Study of live lecture attendance, student perceptions and expectations. Medical Science Educator 2021;31(2):697–707.

36. USMLE Step 1 Transition to Pass/Fail Only Score Reporting. The United States Medical Licensing Examination. 2022. Available at: https://www.usmle.org/usmle-step-1-transition-passfail-only-score-reporting. Accessed June 1, 2022.

37. The American Board of Surgery Continuous Certification Program. The American Board of Surgery. 2022. Available at: https://www.absurgery.org/default.jsp?exam-moc. Accessed 30 July 2022.

38. Martin E. Moore's law is alive and well. Medium. Available at: https://medium.com/predict/moores-law-is-alive-and-well-eaa49a450188. Accessed July 26, 2022.

39. Hashimoto DA, Rosman G, Rus D, Meireles OR. Artificial intelligence in surgery: promises and perils. Ann Surg 2018;268(1):70–6.

40. Blease C, Kaptchuk TJ, Bernstein MH, Mandl KD, Halamka JD, DesRoches CM. Artificial intelligence and the future of primary care: exploratory qualitative study of UK general practitioners' views. J Med Internet Res 2019;21(3):e12802.

41. Williams VN, Medina J, Medina A, Clifton S. Bridging the millennial generation expectation gap: perspectives and strategies for physician and interprofessional faculty. Am J Med Sci 2017;353(2):109–15.

42. Wallace J. Work commitment in the legal profession: a study of Baby Boomers and Generation Xers. International Journal of the Legal Profession 2006;13(2):137–51.

43. Oblinger D. The next generation of educational engagement. Journal of Interactive Media in Education 2004;8.

44. Roberts DH, Newman LR, Schwartzstein RM. Twelve tips for facilitating Millennials' learning. Med Teach 2012;34(4):274–8.

45. Price C. Why Don't my students think i'm groovy?: The new "R"s for engaging millennial learners. The Teaching Professor; 2009.

Machine Learning and Artificial Intelligence in Surgical Research

Shruthi Srinivas, MD[a], Andrew J. Young, MD[b],*

KEYWORDS

• Machine learning • Surgical research • Artificial intelligence

KEY POINTS

- Machine learning (ML), a branch of artificial intelligence involving teaching a computer to read and interpret data, is a tool that can be used for prediction in medical and surgical research.
- ML depends on a variety of traditional research metrics to achieve optimal predictions and to generate reproducible research.
- Avenues of current and future research include diagnostics, operative decision-making, operative time prediction, and surgical education.

BACKGROUND

Machine learning (ML), a branch of artificial intelligence, involves the development of algorithms focused on pattern recognition and learning for computer-based prediction, and has developed over the past two decades as an important tool within the field of medicine and medical research. As it becomes more successful, applicable, and useful within medicine, its applications to the surgical subspecialties have become clear as well.

Branches of Machine Learning

Traditional ML as it is understood today was first developed in the 1950s and 1960s, at which point it was mainly generated in three branches: symbolic learning as described by Hunt and colleagues, statistical methodology as described by Nilsson and colleagues, and neural networks as described by Rosenblatt and colleagues[1–3] Over the subsequent 50 years, advances developed in each theory, allowing for more direct applicability to the field of medicine and, subsequently surgery. Now, ML is principally

[a] Department of Surgery, The Ohio State University, 370 West 9th Avenue, Columbus, OH 43210, USA; [b] Division of Trauma, Critical Care, and Burn, The Ohio State University, 181 Taylor Avenue, Suite 1102K, Columbus, OH 43203, USA
* Corresponding author.
E-mail address: Andrew.Young@osumc.edu

Surg Clin N Am 103 (2023) 299–316
https://doi.org/10.1016/j.suc.2022.11.002
0039-6109/23/© 2022 Elsevier Inc. All rights reserved.

understood in three sections: supervised learning, unsupervised learning, and rein-forcement learning.[4]

Supervised learning

Supervised learning, often regarded as the most basic of ML algorithms, involves teaching a computer to match pairs. For example, a computer can be shown a set of photos labeled "dog" versus "cat" and can learn to identify dogs versus cats in sub-sequent images. This involves both classification and regression, depending on whether a class label or a number is generated. It also involves decision trees, in which decision-making proceeds is mimicked by a computer, and Bayesian models, in which prior probabilities are used to estimate future outcomes.[5] The major drawback of this model is that the computer needs to be taught how to interpret further images, scenarios, or patient classifications.

Unsupervised learning

Unsupervised learning involves the computer generating its own rules for the identifi-cation and classification of systems.[6] Most frequently described as "clustering", this involves the computer taking on a set of data independently and sorting based on an identified factor. Although this decreases the need for user interaction, it also is prone to error. For example, if a computer is asked to sort a group of shapes, whereas the intended outcome may be sets of circles, triangles, and squares, the computer may instead sort based on color, when not prompted by the intended user.

Reinforcement learning

In reinforcement learning, the computer is trained to interact with its environment to generate a result that is most favorable to it.[7] As an optimal outcome is approached, the computer is rewarded, which helps drive future decisions toward similar out-comes. If the computer makes an error, it receives a penalty, which also leads back toward the correct or most optimal outcome and is learned for future iterations of the same or similar problems.

DISCUSSION
History of Machine Learning in Medicine

The arguments for use of ML in medicine are plenty.[8] Hospital systems are built to collect large volumes of patient information with clear data on diagnosis, treatment, prognosis, and outcomes; these data can be harnessed beyond the scope of a single individual or team to make predictions on subsequent diagnostic dilemmas. This world of personalized medicine allows for the ultimate in crowd-sourcing—under-standing the experiences of millions to inform the care of one. New diagnoses such as coronary artery disease, traumatic rib fractures, and new pancreatic cancer can be managed in accordance with globally agreed-upon standards of care, as opposed to treatment per provider experience or preference, and can reflect therapy tailored to specific patient criteria.[9] Medical errors such as overdoses, allergies and cross-reactivity between medications, and duplicate medications, could be decreased by application of ML, allowing computers to analyze the millions of interactions between various medications and preventing inaccuracies.[10] Patients with complicated diag-noses who seek out health care in a variety of forms (inpatient, outpatient, consulting services, various hospital systems) could have their care centralized and standard-ized, and this could allow for more rapid detection of patterns that ultimately lead to diagnosis, treatment, and recovery.[11,12]

While enticing, and certainly applicable, the world of ML has interfaced within med-icine for only a short period of time. This was first alluded to in 1970, at which time the rise in medical knowledge generated concerns about the gap between physician knowledge and needed knowledge, proposing the use of computer technology to bridge that gap.[13] At this time, computed technology was used for basic tasks, such as interpretation of electrocardiograms, and was considered a threat to specialized fields of medicine such as anesthesiology, radiology, and pathology.[14] As the field of medicine has had growth, ML has grown of interest to individuals without as much experience, prompting many primers that strive to educate practicing physicians about the benefits and drawbacks of incorporating ML into daily practice.[15,16] ML algorithms and applications remain an area of fruitful research for which an understanding is critical in advancing clinical knowledge in medicine and surgery.

Supervised learning

Initially discussed as "symbolic learning" by Hunt and colleagues, supervised learning was first described as the "Concept Learning System" (CLS) in which the computer was used to understand large sections of data. Computers were taught a concept, such as "bird" versus "non-bird" and were able to generate lists within data sets matching each category. In plotting variables against one another, the computer was able to generate patterns that could be interpreted by human researchers. In the 1980s, these developed into programs that understood advanced classification schemes and tapped into extensive domain knowledge by information specialists; however, at this time, these systems remained only able to perform what they were programmed to do without demonstrating the capacity for true learning.

In the early 1990s, symbolic learning changed with the demonstration of the Iterative Dichotomizer 3 (ID3) algorithm as described by Quinlan, and the subsequent application of such to diagnose soybean diseases with accuracy by Michalski.[17,18] This was the first demonstration of decision trees, supervised ML algorithms in which the computer encounters a series of decisions, known as nodes, and plot a route to the correct outcome. For example, in the diagnosis of sepsis, there are several laboratory results and vital signs that trend clinicians towards or away from this diagnosis.[16] Symbolic learning in the form of decision trees, neural networks, and random forest modeling represents an overarching concept in which the computer learns to follow these values in a similar path to a clinician to make a diagnosis with similar information.

Over the subsequent decades, symbolic learning has become more frequently used in medicine. Given its ability to mimic a physician's diagnostic thought process, it has been studied in several diagnostic and prognostic challenges, including, but not limited to, diagnosis of breast cancer, oncology, and cirrhosis.[19–21] Further success was found in the generation of the RELIEF algorithm and its descendants, which allows for the assignment of relevance to each variable within the decision tree—for example, a sepsis predictive algorithm could place more weight on leukocytosis than on anemia, and so on.[22,23] Generation of these features made algorithms more human-like, and thus more applicable to medical decision-making and diagnosis in general.[24,25]

In addition, medical research has grown through the naïve Bayes classifier, a probabilistic model that predicts outcomes based on the relative probability of various options with prior knowledge.[5,26] For example, in the previously discussed model on sepsis, a naïve Bayes classifier would predict that a patient with a profound leukocytosis would be more likely to have sepsis as several previous patients with leukocytosis were also more likely to have sepsis. In recent years, there have been developments to Bayesian models in the form of variants. The m-variant, described by Cestnik, showed improved outcomes as compared with the naïve Bayesian model in similar medical prognosis situations.[27] A recursive structure has also been developed that allows for the utilization of naïve Bayesian predictive models within decision trees, which is more ideal within the practice of medicine.[28] Overall, supervised learning remains one of the highest used areas of ML within the practice of medicine.

Unsupervised learning

In contrast to supervised ML models, unsupervised learning has had later incorporation into medical research. Given the breadth of available patient data, which worsened with the generation of the electronic medical record, analyzing data has become more difficult due to challenges with size and computing power. One such example is neural networks that involve the generation of thousands of parameters to closely approximate actual human decision-making. These can be used in both supervised and unsupervised ML. Owing to their expansive requirements, a neural network cannot be comprehended by the human brain and lacks in transparency.[29] An early limitation was the inability to follow non-linear pathways, although this expanded after the generation of activation functions within algorithms.[30] Although modeling is accurate, the inability of the end user to understand the algorithm's steps and sequences limits the ability to learn from the models, which in health care, limits the ability of the practicing physician or the researcher to draw meaningful conclusions from the application of these networks.[31] The future in neural network lies in developing some transparency to the model system; although advances have been made, this remains the area of most potential.[32] In recent years, natural language processing has become more well-studied, which involves ML within the electronic health record to parse coding and diagnosis information.[33] Image recognition is also a big area of further research, involving the application of neural networks to understand both radiographical and pathological images for more accurate and rapid diagnosis.[34]

Reinforcement learning

Studied primarily in game theory, reinforcement learning is the latest branch of ML to become applicable to the world of medicine, with growth in the past decade. Initial applications were in dynamic treatment regimes, which involve sequential decisions to generate personalized management based on patient factors, response to therapy, and covariate history.[35] These often involve models known as Q-functions and have been studied in sarcoma, psychiatry, and human immunodeficiency virus.[36–38] Reinforcement learning represents one of the most quickly growing areas of ML research in medicine.

Research Metrics in Machine Learning

ML technologies can be applied to many different problems, such as cohort mapping, natural language processing, and imaging processing, as described above. Though not often thought of as an ML algorithm, logistic regression is a tool of all surgical research that is vital to the generation of strong ML algorithms, and the concept of p-value is often used to determine statistical significance of the algorithm. Although one example of an important research metric, there are many other metrics that can impact the generation and use of ML algorithms.

Sensitivity/specificity

Sensitivity is the ability of a test to correctly identify patients with a disease. It can be calculated by dividing the number of true positives by the number of true positives plus the number of false negatives (total number of patients with the disease). Specificity is the ability of a test to correctly identify people without the disease. It can be calculated by dividing the total number of true negatives by the number of false positives (total number of patients without the disease). This information may be critical when evaluating new ML algorithms to implement within a health care system.[39] The risk of missing a diagnosis (eg, the risk of missing a stroke) versus the cost of false positives (eg, the cost of a head CT for every patient that screens positive in the algorithm being evaluated), is a key deciding factor for use and adoption of any prediction algorithm. For example, in generating a preoperative neurosurgical diagnosis, sensitivity and specificity is key to accurately predicting preoperative diagnosis, which informs surgical planning and preoperative risk.[40]

Accuracy

The general term accuracy is used to describe the closeness of a measurement to the true value, or the number of cases decided correctly. For binary classifiers (disease present or not present), accuracy refers to the statistical measure of how well a binary classification test correctly identifies the outcome. Mathematically, it is the proportion of correct predictions (both true positives and true negatives) among the total number of cases evaluated. Thus, it is a single number that can sum up both sensitivity and specificity.[41] This metric can be helpful when evaluating the merits of an ML prediction model. Although there may be superior metrics to use, this metric is well understood within the medical community. In plastic surgery, for example, diagnostic accuracy allows clinicians to model surgical intervention and compare to clinician outcomes to assess for future desirability.[42]

Positive predictive value/negative predictive value

Positive predictive value and negative predictive value are considered conditional probabilities within research because they rely upon the condition of the test being either positive or negative. These are not considered intrinsic to the to the test as they depend on the prevalence of the characteristic being tested for. Like accuracy, this is generally a well-understood metric that can be used to determine important differences in prediction algorithms when evaluating which algorithm to use in a health care setting. Predictive values are helpful in biomarker-based systems that analyze risk factors for surgery and for postoperative complications.[43]

Discrimination

Discrimination refers to how well a model differentiates between high-risk individuals having an event and low-risk individuals not having an event. Discrimination can be measured numerically using the area under the receiver operator curve, or c statistic.

The concordance (c) statistic is the most commonly used performance measure to indicate the discriminative ability of generalized linear regression models. For a binary outcome, the c-statistic is identical to the area under the receiver operating curve (ROC). Thus, it is frequently reported for prediction models. The c statistic and area under the ROC convey useful information, yet do not fill in all possible gaps when evaluating a prediction model.[44] ROC is independent of decision threshold, which is both advantageous and disadvantageous. It can reflect which test is more accurate but fails to recognize that accuracy may vary based on the population of study. Importantly, it performs poorly with imbalanced data.[45] The ROC is a representation of true positive false positive fractions, both of which are independent of disease prevalence; hence the ROC also does not depend on prevalence. The various operating points on the ROC curve can have different meaning depending on the prevalence of the disease, the cost of the test, the cost of missing true positive patients, and the cost of false positive patients. Discrimination models have been shown in specific situations, such as cardiac surgery, to produce more optimal modeling outcomes compared with traditional logistic regression.[46]

Calibration

Calibration is a measure of how well the predicted probabilities agree with actual observed risk.

This measures the degree to which the predicted probabilities match the actual observed risk.[47] Interestingly, calibration can vary depending on a patient's risk. For example, a hospital system is evaluating a new fall-risk model that overall has mediocre calibration but performs superbly when patients have a fall-risk between 20% and 80%. Despite what appears to be average performance, nursing leadership indicates keen interest in a model such as this because staff can easily identify patients who are at very high and very low risk of falling. Those patients who have a mix of risk factors that remain in an uncertain fall-risk category. In this example, a calibration graph is ideal for visualizing this relationship.

Hosmer–Lemeshow statistic

Originally described in 1980, the Hosmer–Lemeshow statistic directly compares the average predicted risk of a study group to the proportion that actually develops the disease. The model returns p values, with higher (closer to 1) indicating a better "fit".[48] One downside to this test is that it does not take the problem of overfitting into account. Overfitting is observed when an ML algorithm is developed that predicts the training data too well, so exposure to new data causes the algorithm to perform poorly. In the world of surgical research, limiting overfitting remains an area of active research, as this is often a limiting factor in many models, including endocrine surgery and ovarian surgery.[49,50] The test also does not give any guidance on the number of subgroups, g, which is usually calculated by taking the number of covariates in the model and adding 1. Changing g can lead to significant differences in the p values.[51]

Brier score

The Brier Score, considered a proper scoring rule, takes into account calibration as well as sharpness (the concentration of predictive distribution).[52,53] A proper scoring rule is one in which the forecaster/model is rewarded for giving an honest answer and not one that is hedged. For example, if a disease occurs roughly 95% of the time, a model may look to have favorable characteristics if it predicts the presence of disease 100% of the time. However, this model would have a poor Brier score because the prediction distribution would be incorrect. The Brier score for a model can range from 0 for a perfect model to 0.25 for a noninformative model with a 50% incidence of the outcome. Like the mean squared error (MSE), this captures both calibration and discrimination aspects.[52,54] Like all models, it can be used for a variety of surgical research goals.

Mean squared error/root mean squared error

Both metrics have been widely used to measure model performance in the literature and both are considered proper error metrics. Root mean squared error (RMSE) has been suggested to not be a good indicator of average model performance; however, there remains much debate.[55,56] RMSE is more appropriate when the errors follow a normal distribution (Gaussian), whereas MSE is optimal for Laplacian errors.[57] However, both can be useful depending on the goal of the prediction model. For example, in tests attempting to predict length of the operative course, using RMSE can more accurately model.[58] The ability to use elements of both discrimination and calibration in a single number is the underlying success of this model.

Net reclassification

This model involves classifying patients in risk categories and determining new models perform compared with previous models. Risk differences are classified based on the actual outcomes patients experienced (ie having vs not having the event of interest such as death or a stroke).[59] Recent data use net reclassification to quantify surgical complexity.[60]

Other performance measures

This list is not exhaustive but offers a glimpse into important error metrics that are critical in building and evaluating prediction models. Other performance metrics include, but are not limited to, Akaike Information Criterion, Bayesian Index, decision curve analysis, integrated discrimination improvement, scaled Brier score, log loss, and F1 score.[61–63]

Reproducible Research

Reproducible research is the gold standard for which scientific claims can be verified within the scientific community.[64] When evaluating a study that uses standard statistical techniques, statistical significance is denoted with the p value, and it is generally assumed that the statistics could be reasonably reproduced with a similar study design. This assumption has worked well for the medical community until the use of more complex statistical techniques like ML with the ever-growing ML techniques, the ability to reasonably reproduce research becomes almost impossible. This is in part due to the complexity of the code associated with producing algorithms, but it also in part due to the inherent "black box" nature of many ML algorithms.[65] The black box paradigm refers to the inability for anyone, including those that constructed the algorithm, to understand why the computer is arriving at the answer it does.[66] An artificial neural net is a classic example of this problem.[67]

Data pipeline

The various stages of a study can be broken down into study design, data collection, data tidying, statistical evaluation, summary statistics, and reporting of statistically significant findings (p value). Areas within the study that typically have little oversight include the summary statistics, how the data are collected, how the raw data are tidied, what is done with missing values, and variations on which variations in the statistical models are used. These stages are referred to as the "data pipeline." A data pipeline in ML is considered a useful technique to efficiently move data between one step in the model-building algorithm to the next to ensure that the inputs of the previous step in the pipeline accurately match the inputs of the next step.[68] Interestingly, although there is much debate and concentration on study design and the conclusions of a study (p value), there is little debate over the areas of the data pipeline despite each presenting a risk of introduction of bias and decreasing the possibility of reproducibility.[69]

Rise of the Standardized Tool

The issues surrounding ML algorithms notwithstanding, the concerns regarding the quality of published medical research has grown in the last 20 years as the volume of published research has increased substantially.[70] Although there was recognition within the literature as early as the 1930s regarding the poor quality of published research, there has not been a concerted effort devoted to improving quality until recently.[71,72] With increasing recognition of the problem, the CONsolidated Standards Of Reporting Trials (CONSORT) Statement was published.[73] CONSORT focused on reporting of clinical trials, and while thought to be initially successful there was much room for improvement. Thus began the global push toward standardizing many aspects of medical experiments.

Transparent Reporting of a Multivariable Prediction Model for Individual Prognosis or Diagnosis

The reproducibility problem was recognized by The Transparent Reporting of a multivariable prediction model for Individual Prognosis or Diagnosis (TRIPOD) Initiative. In 2015, the TRIPOD Statement was published in the Annals of Internal Medicine that described a checklist of 22 items that were essential for transparent reporting of a prediction model study.[74] Authors of prediction studies were encouraged to include a completed 23-item checklist along with the study findings. The checklist touches on every major section of reported study including the title, abstract, introduction, methods, results, and discussion. The list is comprehensive, but it still leaves wide gaps in interpretation of the requirements. For example, the only required item for evaluating model performance is including confidence intervals with performance measures.

Prediction Model Risk of Bias Assessment Tool

Another framework that is available called the Prediction model Risk of Bias Assessment Tool (PROBAST) can be used for appraisal of prediction models.[75] Originally designed for systematic reviews, the tool walks the user through a four-step process including (1) specifying the systematic review question, (2) classifying the type of prediction model, (3) assessing the risk of bias, and then summing up the findings of each previous step in to an (4) overall judgment of bias and applicability. This tool provides a standardized methodology for researchers designing prediction algorithms, ML-based or otherwise. Furthermore, it aids in guideline creation, article reviews, and organizations seeking to evaluate potential prediction models for use within a health care system.

Machine Learning in Surgical Research

Overall, ML in its three major forms has developed significantly since inception 50 years ago. As a predictive software by nature, applications in medicine and surgery remain strong. Early ML research showed success primarily in the ability of pattern recognition to be applicable to large datasets, alleviating the burden of individual researcher-based analysis of whole databases.[76] Initial forms of data mining then developed in sophistication over time to meet needs, and now more accurately address scalability and efficacy, cleaning of complicated data sets via removal of noise, and involvement of end user in "interactive" data mining.[77–79]

As ML has become more commonplace in medicine and surgery, many unique challenges have arisen.[8,80] Applying computer-based algorithms to patient data calls into question concerns regarding patient privacy and ownership of data.[81] In addition, medical terminology can be extremely heterogeneous, with similar conditions described in multiple ways based on most recent coding, hospital preference, and physician practice. This makes generating consistent variables challenging. Related to surgical fields specifically, applications of ML lie in diagnosis and prognosis, intraoperative decision-making, predictions on operations including time and technique, and skill development, teaching, and resident education.[82,83] As ML grows in incorporation in the day-to-day clinical practice of surgeons, its role in clinical and translational research also grows to match.

Preoperative diagnosis and prognosis

Perhaps the easiest area of understanding in the applicability of ML to surgical practice is preoperative diagnosis. Given the inherent applicability of predictive modeling to diagnosis, this remains an area of strong interest in surgical modeling. Much of this comes from the world of trauma surgery, a field highly structured on algorithms, protocols, and modeling.[84] Early papers were used in penetrating injuries to predict survivability, using neural networks to extrapolate based on Revised Trauma Score, Injury Severity Score, and several other easily available metrics in the trauma bay.[67,85] Statistical modeling was used to weight factors that affected discharge disposition in trauma patients, and models were generated using eight separate variables to identify which of these, often frailty index, provided the most predictive value in learning which trauma patients die after presentation to the emergency department.[86,87] Further research within the world of trauma has recently focused on niche preoperative factors such as weather, in-flight bleeding scores in helicopter transport, early recognition of acute kidney injury, and predictors of early mortality in traumatic brain injury patients.[88–91] The generation of these accurate and rapidly applicable models allows for the identification of worrisome patients early and quickly in the clinical course—sometimes even before their arrival in the trauma bay—which allows for more rapid assessment and appropriate therapy, theoretically improving survival.

Although trauma represents the most tangible applicability of predictive modeling, the same advantages of diagnostics have been analyzed outside of the trauma bay as well. ML remains beneficial in analyzing patient's preoperative risk, with studies that are curated to individual databases outperforming traditional databases in predicting surgical complications and death.[92–94] Models have also been generated that describe prognostic nuances such as opioid use after surgery and likelihood of postoperative acute kidney injury.[95,96] Overall, this allows for a form of personalized medicine that is curated and individualized, and represents a promising future direction of health care.

As ML has developed over time, a critical development has been the ability to teach computers to interpret radiographical images for precise, rapid, and goal-focused diagnosis in the trauma bay. Two areas of intense study have been in identifying orthopedic injuries[97–99] and in managing rib fractures,[100,101] and represent areas of future growth in ML within the trauma population.

Operative decision-making

ML has also been studied in its role in affecting intraoperative decision-making. Studies in decision-making are varied. Some affect preoperative decision-making, such as imaging studies more capable of diagnosing hiatal hernias preoperatively, and predictive models that use deep learning to identify gastric cancer patients at risk of D1 versus D2 lymphadenopathy requiring more extensive resection.[102,103] Within the operating room, ML algorithms have been studied that can, in real-time, identify patients at risk of developing intraoperative hypoxemia or hypotension, which can affect operative healing, outcomes, and ultimately patient survival.[104,105] These studies aim to identify patients at high risk of developing these comorbidities to allow for earlier correction, which prevents untimely complications during critical portions of the procedure.

Neurosurgical research and spine surgery are areas of interest in terms of intraoperative decision-making; algorithms have been developed that analyze various preoperative conditions and apply operative interventions to patient scenarios to understand which operation might give patients the best outcome.[106,107] Studies on healthy subjects within plastic surgery generated a repository of normal faces on which operative interventions can be simulated with ML, allowing for an understanding of postoperative outcomes that helps surgeons plan operative intervention into injured faces.[108] Multiple studies on oncology subjects, including within otolaryngology and breast cancer, have been applied retrospectively to analyze margins of surgical specimens for adequacy.[109,110] Although few studies have studied this clinically in real time, with advancement, these may represent the future of intraoperative ML.[111] Again, this all supports a future of personalized medicine that draws on the experience of many patients to support one in a way that a human researcher cannot imagine of providing care.

Operative predictions: time and technique

In addition to preoperative planning, decision-making, and identification of patients who require early operative intervention, a major area of research combining ML and surgical management arises in the world of operative optimization. It is known that longer operative times correlate with poorer outcomes; in addition, knowledge of operative times is essential at the administrative level for appropriate case planning, resource allocation, and, ultimately, improved cost.[58] Multiple studies have analyzed repositories of case logs to determine more accurate case timing, which allows for improved surgical planning, ultimately affecting patient and provider time in the operating room to allowed for improved utilization.[112–114] Studies have also extensively studied operating room efficiency, including identifying surgeries with high risk of cancellation, managing in real time the operating room and postanesthesia care units, and, in the era of coronavirus disease-2019, ML was applied to optimize the efficiency of operating room booking time and reduce nursing overtime to save hospital cost.[115,116]

Skill development, teaching, and resident education

Finally, ML represents a unique opportunity for progression of surgical education through skills practice, teaching, and education of resident physicians. Although somewhat at an early stage of practice, ML has been shown to be a useful tool in assessing competence of residents for independent practice.[117–119] This not only allows for stratification of residents and identification of knowledge gaps, but also allows for generation of objective criteria that differentiate expert surgeons from novice surgeons, allowing for the development of medical education curriculum geared towards training more competent surgeons. ML has also been studied in improving faculty evaluations of resident physicians and for the development of coaching strategies for trainees.[120,121] ML also has application in evolving surgical resident skills, supporting integration into the operative environment to identify areas of correction in real-time and promote higher efficiency, especially as resident training continues to involve minimally invasive operations such as robotic and laparoscopic surgery.[122–124]

SUMMARY

Overall, ML has evolved continually since its inception in the mid-1950s, with broad-reaching implications across the fields of medicine and surgery. As the three arms of ML continue to evolve and accommodate the needs of surgical research, they allow for growth in the field of personalized surgery, ultimately improving patient, provider, and hospital outcomes. Although surgical primers have accelerated the ability for the novel surgeon or researcher to use ML, the specific principles and practice of ML and artificial intelligence remain a large area of growth. There are many frameworks that allow constructing and evaluating reproducible research. In addition, there are software tools that improve access and sharing of methods in ML algorithm construction. Communities such as Kaggle and Hackernoon allow discussion of methodology used and cross-talk between medical and nonmedical communities alike.[125,126] Thus, despite the increasing complexity and volume of ML algorithms, there are new tools to help ensure that research remains attainable and reproducible.

CLINICS CARE POINTS

- Machine learning is an evolving area of research and clinical practice in surgery and surgical research.
- As ML continues to grow and become more accessible to individual surgeons, understanding and reproducibility are key to ensuring future success.

DISCLOSURE

The authors have nothing to disclose.

REFERENCES

1. Hunt EB, Marin J, Stone PJ. Experiments in induction. Academic Press. 1966. Available at: https://psycnet.apa.org/record/1966-08232-000. Accessed July 10, 2022.
2. Nilsson NJ. Learning Machines: Foundations of Trainable Pattern-Classifying Systems. McGraw-Hill. 1965. Available at: https://openlibrary.org/books/OL5908236M/Learning_machines. Accessed July 10, 2022.
3. Rosenblatt F. Principles of Neurodynamics: Perceptrons and the Theory of Brain Mechanisms. Spartan Books. 1962. Available at: https://books.google.com/books/about/Principles_of_Neurodynamics.html?id=7FhRAAAAMAAJ. Accessed July 10, 2022.
4. Mahesh B. Machine Learning Algorithms - A Review. Int J Sci Res 2018. https://doi.org/10.21275/ART20203995.
5. Spiegelhalter D, Dawid A, Lauritzen S, et al. 1993 undefined. Bayesian analysis in expert systems. JSTOR. Available at: https://www.jstor.org/stable/2245959?casa_token=vopHuwlK5bYAAAAA:_NZQ31tkl3EaM5IVRnKX7huleyDNaztUIGDJw_PzV7Hcx_d0RZPeb2HdACROEax3l1VNbsTSB-P_m_WriMNsmhN-uSLLR3Qz_NQ0klqCidYoJKC-5aY. Accessed July 10, 2022.
6. Ghahramani Z. Unsupervised Learning. 2004. Available at: http://www.gatsby.ucl.ac.uk/~zoubin. Accessed July 13, 2022.
7. Sutton R, Barto A. Reinforcement learning: an introduction. 2nd ed. MIT Press; 2018. Available at: http://incompleteideas.net/book/the-book-2nd.html. Accessed July 13, 2022.
8. Rajkomar A, Dean J, Kohane I. Machine learning in medicine. N Engl J Med 2019;380(14):1347–58.
9. Bertsimas D, Orfanoudaki A, Weiner RB. Personalized treatment for coronary artery disease patients: a machine learning approach. Health Care Manag Sci 2020;23(4):482–506.
10. Institute of Medicine. *To err is human: building a safer health system*. Washington, DC: The National Academies Press; 2000.
11. Richens JG, Lee CM, Johri S. Improving the accuracy of medical diagnosis with causal machine learning. Nat Commun 2020;11(1):1–9.
12. Schaefer J, Lehne M, Schepers J, et al. The use of machine learning in rare diseases: a scoping review. Orphanet J Rare Dis 2020;15(1):1–10.
13. Schwartz WB. Medicine and the computer. N Engl J Med 2010;283(23):1257–64.
14. Schläpfer J, Wellens HJ. Computer-Interpreted Electrocardiograms: benefits and Limitations. J Am Coll Cardiol 2017;70(9):1183–92.

15. Waljee AK, Higgins PDR. Machine learning in medicine: a primer for physicians. Am J Gastroenterol 2010;105(6):1224–6.
16. Lammers DT, Eckert CM, Ahmad MA, et al. A surgeon's guide to machine learning. Ann Surg 2021;1–5. https://doi.org/10.1097/AS9.0000000000000091.
17. Michalski R. Learning by being told and learning from examples: An experimental comparison of the two methods of knowledge acquisition. Int J Policy Anal Inf Syst 1980;4(2). Available at: http://www.mli.gmu.edu/papers/79-80/80-2.pdf. Accessed July 10, 2022.
18. Quinlan J. Discovering Rules from Large Collections of Examples: A Case Study. Edinburgh University Press. 1979. Available at: https://cir.nii.ac.jp/crid/1572261550282070144. Accessed July 10, 2022.
19. Elomaa T, Holsti N. An experimental comparison of inducing decision trees and decision lists in noisy domains. Proceedings of the Fourth European Working Session on Learning. 1989. Available at: https://researchportal.tuni.fi/en/publications/an-experimental-comparison-of-inducing-decision-trees-and-decisio. Accessed July 10, 2022.
20. Lesmo L, Saitta L, Torasso P. Learning of fuzzy production rules for medical diagnosis. Approximate Reasoning Decis Anal 1993;901–12. https://doi.org/10.1016/B978-1-4832-1450-4.50095-X.
21. Cestnik B, Kononenko I, Bratko I. ASSISTANT 86: a knowledge-elicitation tool for sophisticated users. Proceedings of the 2nd European Conference on European Working Session on Learning. Published online 1987. Accessed July 10, 2022. https://dl.acm.org/doi/abs/10.5555/3108739.3108742
22. Kononenko I. Estimating attributes: Analysis and extensions of RELIEF. Lecture Notes Computer Sci (including subseries Lecture Notes Artif Intelligence Lecture Notes Bioinformatics) 1994;784 LNCS:171–82.
23. Urbanowicz RJ, Meeker M, la Cava W, et al. Relief-based feature selection: introduction and review. J Biomed Inform 2018;85:189–203.
24. Zhu F, Li X, Tang H, et al. Machine learning for the preliminary diagnosis of dementia. Scientific Programming 2020;2020. https://doi.org/10.1155/2020/5629090.
25. Ghosh P, Azam S, Jonkman M, et al. Efficient prediction of cardiovascular disease using machine learning algorithms with relief and lasso feature selection techniques. IEEE Access 2021;9:19304–26.
26. Pompe U, Kononenko I. Probabilistic first-order classification. Lecture Notes in Computer Science (including subseries Lecture Notes in Artificial Intelligence and Lecture Notes in Bioinformatics) 1997;1297:235–42. https://doi.org/10.1007/3540635149_52/COVER/.
27. Artificial BCProc 9th EC on, 1990 undefined. Estimating probabilities: A crucial task in machine learning. ci.nii.ac.jp. Available at: https://ci.nii.ac.jp/naid/10016425442/. Accessed July 10, 2022.
28. Langley P. Induction of recursive bayesian classifiers. Lecture Notes Computer Sci (including subseries Lecture Notes Artif Intelligence Lecture Notes Bioinformatics) 1993;667 LNAI:153–64.
29. Minsky M, Papert S. Perceptrons Cambridge. MIT Press. 1969. Available at: https://scholar.google.com/scholar?q=Minsky%20M.%20In:%20Papert%20S,%20editor.%20Perceptrons.%20Cambridge,%20MA:%20MIT%20Press,%201969. Accessed July 10, 2022.
30. Nwankpa C., Ijomah W., Gachagan A., et al. Activation Functions: Comparison of trends in Practice and Research for Deep Learning. *arXiv181103378*, 2018. https://doi.org/10.48550/arXiv.1811.03378.

31. Ribeiro MT, Singh S, Guestrin C. "Why should i trust you?" Explaining the predictions of any classifier. Proceedings of the ACM SIGKDD International Conference on Knowledge Discovery and Data Mining. 2016;13-17-August-2016:1135-1144. doi:10.1145/2939672.2939778

32. Haykin S, Lippmann R. Neural networks, a comprehensive foundation. Int J Neural Syst 1994;5(4):363–4. Available at: https://scholar.google.com/scholar?q=Haykin%20S.%20Neural%20networks:%20a%20comprehensive%20foundation.%20New%20York:%20Macmillan,%201994.#d=gs_cit&t=1657583311042&u=%2Fscholar%3Fq%3Dinfo%3AT9-pOG_zTdCAJ%3Ascholar.google.com%2F%26output%3Dcite%26scirp%3D0%26hl%3Den. Accessed July 10, 2022.

33. Friedman C, Hripcsak G. Natural Language Processing and Its Future in Medicine. Information Resources. 1999. Available at: http://www.columbia.edu/itc/hs/medinfo/g6080/misc/articles/friedman.pdf. Accessed July 12, 2022.

34. Ker J, Wang L, Rao J, et al. Deep Learning Applications in Medical Image Analysis. IEEE Access 2017;6:9375–9.

35. Alanazi HO, Abdullah AH, Qureshi KN. A Critical Review for Developing Accurate and Dynamic Predictive Models Using Machine Learning Methods in Medicine and Health Care. J Med Syst 2017;41(4):1–10.

36. Thall PF, Wathen JK. Covariate-adjusted adaptive randomization in a sarcoma trial with multi-stage treatments. Stat Med 2005;24(13):1947–64.

37. Murphy SA, Oslin DW, Rush AJ, et al. Methodological Challenges in Constructing Effective Treatment Sequences for Chronic Psychiatric Disorders. Neuropsychopharmacology 2006;32(2):257–62, 2007 32:2.

38. Yu C, Dong Y, Liu J, et al. Incorporating causal factors into reinforcement learning for dynamic treatment regimes in HIV. BMC Med Inform Decis Mak 2019;19(2):19–29.

39. Bossuyt PM, Reitsma JB, Bruns DE, et al. STARD 2015: an updated list of essential items for reporting diagnostic accuracy studies. BMJ 2015;351. https://doi.org/10.1136/BMJ.H5527.

40. Buchlak QD, Esmaili N, Leveque JC, et al. Machine learning applications to clinical decision support in neurosurgery: an artificial intelligence augmented systematic review. Neurosurg Rev 2020;43(5):1235–53.

41. Metz CE. Basic principles of ROC analysis. Semin Nucl Med 1978;8(4):283–98.

42. Mantelakis A, Assael Y, Sorooshian P, et al. Machine Learning Demonstrates High Accuracy for Disease Diagnosis and Prognosis in Plastic Surgery. Plast Reconstr Surg Glob Open 2021;9(6). https://doi.org/10.1097/GOX.0000000000003638.

43. Lötsch J, Ultsch A, Kalso E. Prediction of persistent post-surgery pain by preoperative cold pain sensitivity: biomarker development with machine-learning-derived analysis. BJA: Br J Anaesth 2017;119(4):821–9.

44. Fawcett T. An introduction to ROC analysis. Pattern Recognition Lett 2006;27(8):861–74.

45. Carrington AM, Fieguth PW, Qazi H, et al. A new concordant partial AUC and partial c statistic for imbalanced data in the evaluation of machine learning algorithms. BMC Med Inform Decis Mak 2020;20(1):1–12.

46. Benedetto U, Dimagli A, Sinha S, et al. Machine learning improves mortality risk prediction after cardiac surgery: Systematic review and meta-analysis. J Thorac Cardiovasc Surg 2022;163(6):2075–87.e9.

47. Hilden J, Habbema JDF, Bjerregaard B. The measurement of performance in probabilistic diagnosis. II. Trustworthiness of the exact values of the diagnostic probabilities. Methods Inf Med 1978;17(4):227–37.

48. Hosmer DW, Lemeshow S. Goodness of fit tests for the multiple logistic regression model. Commun Stat - Theor Methods 1980;9(10):1043–69.

49. Staartjes VE, Serra C, Muscas G, et al. Utility of deep neural networks in predicting gross-total resection after transsphenoidal surgery for pituitary adenoma: a pilot study. Neurosurg Focus 2018;45(5):E12.

50. Barber EL, Garg R, Persenaire C, et al. Natural language processing with machine learning to predict outcomes after ovarian cancer surgery. Gynecol Oncol 2021;160(1):182–6.

51. Hosmer DW, Nils LH. Goodness-of-fit processes for logistic regression: Simulation results. Stat Med 2002;21(18):2723–38.

52. Rufibach K. Use of Brier score to assess binary predictions. J Clin Epidemiol 2010;63(8):938–9.

53. Gneiting T, Raftery AE. Strictly Proper Scoring Rules, Prediction, and Estimation. J Am Stat Assoc 2007. https://doi.org/10.1198/016214506000001437.

54. Redelmeier DA, Bloch DA, Hickam DH. Assessing predictive accuracy: how to compare Brier scores. J Clin Epidemiol 1991;44(11):1141–6.

55. Chai T, Draxler RR. Root mean square error (RMSE) or mean absolute error (MAE)? -Arguments against avoiding RMSE in the literature. Geoscientific Model Development 2014;7(3):1247–50.

56. Willmott C, Matsuura K. Advantages of the mean absolute error (MAE) over the root mean square error (RMSE) in assessing average model performance on JSTOR. Clim Res 2005;30(1):79–82. Available at: https://www.jstor.org/stable/24869236#metadata_info_tab_contents. Accessed July 30, 2022.

57. Hodson TO. Root-mean-square error (RMSE) or mean absolute error (MAE): when to use them or not. Geoscientific Model Development 2022;15(14):5481–7.

58. Jackson TD, Wannares JJ, Lancaster RT, et al. Does speed matter? the impact of operative time on outcome in laparoscopic surgery. Surg Endosc 2011;25(7):2288–95.

59. Cook NR. Use and Misuse of the Receiver Operating Characteristic Curve in Risk Prediction. Circulation 2007;115(7):928–35.

60. van Esbroeck A, Rubinfeld I, Hall B, et al. Quantifying surgical complexity with machine learning: Looking beyond patient factors to improve surgical models. Surgery 2014;156(5):1097–105.

61. Bertrand Pv, Sakamoto Y, Ishiguro M, et al. Akaike Information Criterion Statistics. J R Stat Soc Ser A Stat Soc 1988;151(3):567.

62. Kerr KF, McClelland RL, Brown ER, et al. Evaluating the incremental value of new biomarkers with integrated discrimination improvement. Am J Epidemiol 2011;174(3):364–74.

63. Wu YC, Lee WC. Alternative Performance Measures for Prediction Models. PLOS ONE 2014;9(3):e91249.

64. Laine C, Goodman SN, Griswold ME, et al. Reproducible research: moving toward research the public can really trust. Ann Intern Med 2007;146(6):450–3.

65. Chakraborty S, et al. Interpretability of deep learning models: A survey of results," 2017 IEEE SmartWorld. Ubiquitous Intelligence & Computing, Advanced & Trusted Computed, Scalable Computing & Communications, Cloud & Big Data Computing, Internet of People and Smart City Innovation (SmartWorld/

SCALCOM/UIC/ATC/CBDCom/IOP/SCI) 2017;1–6. https://doi.org/10.1109/UIC-ATC.2017.8397411.

66. Ribeiro MT, Singh S, Guestrin C. Model-Agnostic Interpretability of Machine Learning. arxiv 2016. https://doi.org/10.48550/arxiv.1606.05386.

67. DiRusso SM, Sullivan T, Holly C, et al. An artificial neural network as a model for prediction of survival in trauma patients: validation for a regional trauma area. J Trauma 2000;49(2):212–23.

68. 6.1. Pipelines and composite estimators — scikit-learn 1.1.1 documentation. Available at: https://scikit-learn.org/stable/modules/compose.html. Accessed July 30, 2022.

69. Hovy D, Prabhumoye S. Five sources of bias in natural language processing. Lang Linguistics Compass 2021;15(8):e12432.

70. Altman DG, Simera I. A history of the evolution of guidelines for reporting medical research: the long road to the EQUATOR Network. J R Soc Med 2016; 109(2):67–77.

71. Cole L. What is wrong with the medical curriculum? The Lancet 1932;220(5683): 253–4.

72. Schor S, Karten I. Statistical Evaluation of Medical Journal Manuscripts. JAMA 1966;195(13):1123–8.

73. Begg C, Cho M, Eastwood S, et al. Improving the quality of reporting of randomized controlled trials. The CONSORT statement. JAMA 1996;276(8):637–9.

74. Collins GS, Reitsma JB, Altman DG, et al. Transparent reporting of a multivariable prediction model for individual prognosis or diagnosis (TRIPOD): The TRIPOD Statement. BMC Med 2015;13(1):1–10.

75. Wolff RF, Moons KGM, Riley RD, et al. PROBAST: A Tool to Assess the Risk of Bias and Applicability of Prediction Model Studies. Ann Intern Med 2019; 170(1):51–8.

76. Chen MS, Han J, Yu PS. Data mining: An overview from a database perspective. IEEE Trans Knowledge Data Eng 1996;8(6):866–83.

77. Holzinger A, Jurisica I. Knowledge discovery and data mining in biomedical informatics: The future is in integrative, interactive machine learning solutions. Lecture Notes Computer Sci (including subseries Lecture Notes Artif Intelligence Lecture Notes Bioinformatics) 2014;8401:1–18.

78. Xiong H, Pandey G, Steinbach M, et al. Enhancing data analysis with noise removal. IEEE Trans Knowledge Data Eng 2006;18(3):304–19.

79. BlockeelHendrik SM. Scalability and efficiency in multi-relational data mining. ACM SIGKDD Explorations Newsl 2003;5(1):17–30.

80. Cios KJ, William Moore G. Uniqueness of medical data mining. Artif Intelligence Med 2002;26(1–2):1–24.

81. Mooney SJ, Pejaver V. Big data in public health: terminology, machine learning, and privacy. Annu Rev Public Health 2018;39:95.

82. Wang S, Summers RM. Machine learning and radiology. Med Image Anal 2012; 16(5):933–51.

83. Madabhushi A, Lee G. Image analysis and machine learning in digital pathology: Challenges and opportunities. Med Image Anal 2016;33:170–5.

84. Liu NT, Salinas J. Machine learning for predicting outcomes in trauma. Shock 2017. https://doi.org/10.1097/SHK.0000000000000898.

85. Mc Gonigal MD, Cole J, Schwab CW, et al. A new approach to probability of survival scoring for trauma quality assurance. J Trauma 1993;34(6):863–70.

86. Joseph B, Pandit V, Rhee P, et al. Predicting hospital discharge disposition in geriatric trauma patients: Is frailty the answer? J Trauma Acute Care Surg 2013. https://doi.org/10.1097/TA.0b013e3182a833ac.

87. Mitchell RJ, Ting HP, Driscoll T, et al. Identification and internal validation of models for predicting survival and ICU admission following a traumatic injury. Scand J Trauma Resusc Emerg Med 2018;26(1):95. https://doi.org/10.1186/s13049-018-0563-5.

88. Ho VP, Towe CW, Chan J, et al. How's the Weather? Relationship Between Weather and Trauma Admissions at a Level I Trauma Center. World J Surg 2015;39:934–9. https://doi.org/10.1007/s00268-014-2881-8.

89. Yang S, Mackenzie CF, Rock P, et al. Comparison of massive and emergency transfusion prediction scoring systems after trauma with a new Bleeding Risk Index score applied in-flight. J Trauma Acute Care Surg 2021;90(2):268–73.

90. Rashidi HH, Sen S, Palmieri TL, et al. Early Recognition of Burn- and Trauma-Related Acute Kidney Injury: A Pilot Comparison of Machine Learning Techniques. Scientific Rep 2020;10(1):1–9.

91. Amorim RL, Oliveira LM, Malbouisson LM, et al. Prediction of Early TBI Mortality Using a Machine Learning Approach in a LMIC Population. Front Neurol 2020; 10:1366.

92. Ehlers AP, Roy SB, Khor S, et al. Improved risk prediction following surgery using machine learning algorithms. eGEMs 2017;5(2):3.

93. Bihorac A, Ozrazgat-Baslanti T, Ebadi A, et al. MySurgeryRisk: Development and Validation of a Machine-Learning Risk Algorithm for Major Complications and Death after Surgery. Ann Surg 2019;269(4):652.

94. Corey KM, Kashyap S, Lorenzi E, et al. Development and validation of machine learning models to identify high-risk surgical patients using automatically curated electronic health record data (Pythia): A retrospective, single-site study. PLOS Med 2018;15(11):e1002701.

95. Ward A, Jani T, de Souza E, et al. Prediction of Prolonged Opioid Use after Surgery in Adolescents: Insights from Machine Learning. Anesth Analgesia 2021; 133(2):304–13.

96. Li Y, Xu J, Wang Y, et al. A novel machine learning algorithm, Bayesian networks model, to predict the high-risk patients with cardiac surgery-associated acute kidney injury. Clin Cardiol 2020;43(7):752–61.

97. Olczak J, Fahlberg N, Maki A, et al. Artificial intelligence for analyzing orthopedic trauma radiographs: Deep learning algorithms—are they on par with humans for diagnosing fractures? Acta Orthopaedica 2017;88(6):581–6.

98. Choy G, Khalilzadeh O, Michalski M, et al. Current Applications and Future Impact of Machine Learning in Radiology. Radiology 2018;288(2):318.

99. Olthof AW, Shouche P, Fennema EM, et al. Machine learning based natural language processing of radiology reports in orthopaedic trauma. Comput Methods Programs Biomed 2021;208:106304.

100. Weikert T, Noordtzij LA, Bremerich J, et al. Assessment of a Deep Learning Algorithm for the Detection of Rib Fractures on Whole-Body Trauma Computed Tomography. Korean J Radiol 2020;21(7):891.

101. Jin L, Yang J, Kuang K, et al. Deep-learning-assisted detection and segmentation of rib fractures from CT scans: Development and validation of FracNet. eBioMedicine 2020;62:103106.

102. Assaf D, Rayman S, Segev L, et al. Improving pre-bariatric surgery diagnosis of hiatal hernia using machine learning models. Minim Invasive Ther Allied Technol 2021;31(5):760–7.

103. Liu C, Qi L, Feng QX, et al. Performance of a machine learning-based decision model to help clinicians decide the extent of lymphadenectomy (D1 vs. D2) in gastric cancer before surgical resection. Abdom Radiol 2019;44(9):3019–29.

104. Wijnberge M, Geerts BF, Hol L, et al. Effect of a Machine Learning–Derived Early Warning System for Intraoperative Hypotension vs Standard Care on Depth and Duration of Intraoperative Hypotension During Elective Noncardiac Surgery: The HYPE Randomized Clinical Trial. JAMA 2020;323(11):1052–60.

105. Lundberg SM, Nair B, Vavilala MS, et al. Explainable machine-learning predictions for the prevention of hypoxaemia during surgery HHS Public Access Author manuscript. Nat Biomed Eng 2018;2(10):749–60.

106. Saravi B, Hassel F, Ülkümen S, et al. Artificial Intelligence-Driven Prediction Modeling and Decision-making in Spine Surgery Using Hybrid Machine Learning Models. J Personalized Med 2022;12(4):509.

107. Senders JT, Staples PC, Karhade Av, et al. Machine Learning and Neurosurgical Outcome Prediction: A Systematic Review. World Neurosurg 2018;109:476–86.e1.

108. Knoops PGM, Papaioannou A, Borghi A, et al. A machine learning framework for automated diagnosis and computer-assisted planning in plastic and reconstructive surgery. Scientific Rep 2019;9(1):1–12.

109. D'Alfonso TM, Ho DJ, Hanna MG, et al. Multi-magnification-based machine learning as an ancillary tool for the pathologic assessment of shaved margins for breast carcinoma lumpectomy specimens. Mod Pathol 2021;34(8):1487–94.

110. Tighe D, Fabris F, Freitas A. Machine learning methods applied to audit of surgical margins after curative surgery for head and neck cancer. Br J Oral Maxillofac Surg 2021;59(2):209–16.

111. Marsden M, Weyers BW, Bec J, et al. Intraoperative Margin Assessment in Oral and Oropharyngeal Cancer Using Label-Free Fluorescence Lifetime Imaging and Machine Learning. IEEE Trans Biomed Eng 2021;68(3):857–68.

112. Martinez O, Martinez C, Parra CA, et al. Machine learning for surgical time prediction. Comput Methods Programs Biomed 2021;208:106220.

113. Bartek MA, Saxena RC, Solomon S, et al. Improving operating room efficiency: machine learning approach to predict case-time duration. J Am Coll Surg 2019;229(4):346–54.e3.

114. Tuwatananurak JP, Zadeh S, Xu X, et al. Machine learning can improve estimation of surgical case duration: a pilot study. J Med Syst 2019;43(3):1–7.

115. Bellini V, Guzzon M, Bigliardi B, et al. Artificial Intelligence: A New Tool in Operating Room Management. Role of Machine Learning Models in Operating Room Optimization. J Med Syst 2020;44(1):1–10.

116. Rozario N, Rozario D. Can machine learning optimize the efficiency of the operating room in the era of COVID-19? Can J Surg 2020;63(6):E527.

117. Dias RD, Gupta A, Yule SJ. Using machine learning to assess physician competence: a systematic review. Acad Med 2019;94(3):427–39.

118. Winkler-Schwartz A, Bissonnette V, Mirchi N, et al. Artificial intelligence in medical education: best practices using machine learning to assess surgical expertise in virtual reality simulation. J Surg Education 2019;76(6):1681–90.

119. Watson RA. Use of a machine learning algorithm to classify expertise: analysis of hand motion patterns during a simulated surgical task. Acad Med 2014;89(8):1163–7.

120. Thanawala R, Jesneck J, Seymour NE. Novel educational information management platform improves the surgical skill evaluation process of surgical residents. J Surg Education 2018;75(6):e204–11.

121. Rogers MP, DeSantis AJ, Janjua H, et al. The future surgical training paradigm: Virtual reality and machine learning in surgical education. Surgery 2021;169(5):1250–2.

122. Anh NX, Nataraja RM, Chauhan S. Towards near real-time assessment of surgical skills: a comparison of feature extraction techniques. Comput Methods Programs Biomed 2020;187:105234.

123. Wu C, Cha J, Sulek J, et al. Eye-tracking metrics predict perceived workload in robotic surgical skills training. Hum Factors 2020;62(8):1365–86.

124. Ismail Fawaz H, Forestier G, Weber J, et al. Accurate and interpretable evaluation of surgical skills from kinematic data using fully convolutional neural networks. Int J Computer Assisted Radiol Surg 2019;14(9):1611–7.

125. Kaggle. Your Machine Learning and Data Science Community. Available at: https://www.kaggle.com/. Accessed July 31, 2022.

126. HackerNoon - read, write and learn about any technology. Available at: https://hackernoon.com/. Accessed July 31, 2022.

Interpretation and Use of Applied/Operational Machine Learning and Artificial Intelligence in Surgery

Molly J. Douglas, MD[a],*, Rachel Callcut, MD, MSPH[b],
Leo Anthony Celi, MD, MPH, MSc[c,d], Nirav Merchant, BS, MS[e]

KEYWORDS

- Artificial intelligence (AI) • Machine learning (ML) • Computer vision • Prediction
- Deep learning • Computer-aided diagnosis • Augmented reality (AR) • Surgery

KEY POINTS

- Applications for artificial intelligence (AI)/Machine Learning in surgery include image interpretation, data summarization, automated narrative construction, trajectory and risk prediction, and operative navigation and robotics.
- Health-care AI tools are being developed at an exponential pace, outstripping the field's ability to validate and assess them for clinical utility.
- Some AI tools have improved patient care and clinician workflow; yet many algorithms still do not have a defined clinical role.
- Data infrastructure and multidisciplinary teams of clinicians and data scientists will be key in bridging the gap from the algorithm to the bedside.

INTRODUCTION

The work of surgeons is complex, incorporating cognitive and manual skills, analytical processing, creativity, and navigation of nuanced personal interactions. Yet, humans have limitations—we require food and rest, are prone to cognitive biases, are expensive to train, and relative to computers, have a low upper limit for the rate at which new information can be integrated.

[a] Department of Surgery, University of Arizona, 1501 N Campbell Avenue, Tucson, AZ 85724, USA; [b] Trauma, Acute Care Surgery and Surgical Critical Care, University of California, Davis, 2335 Stockton Boulevard, Sacramento, CA 95817, USA; [c] Laboratory of Computational Physiology, Massachusetts Institute of Technology, 77 Massachusetts Avenue, Cambridge, MA 02139, USA; [d] Beth Israel Deaconess Medical Center; [e] Data Science Institute, University of Arizona, 1230 North Cherry Avenue, Tucson, AZ 85721, USA
* Corresponding author.
E-mail address: mjdouglas@arizona.edu
Twitter: @MollyJDouglas (M.J.D.); @callcura (R.C.); @MITCriticalData (L.A.C.)

Surg Clin N Am 103 (2023) 317–333
https://doi.org/10.1016/j.suc.2022.11.004
0039-6109/23/© 2022 Elsevier Inc. All rights reserved.

surgical.theclinics.com

Artificial intelligence (AI) is a branch of computer science using machines to simulate human cognition. It includes machine learning (ML), in which computers recognize patterns from data. AI is unlikely to ever replace surgeons, however, AI tools can be leveraged to support surgeons' workflow and augment decision-making. In this review, we highlight existing uses for AI in the surgical fields and discuss several illustrative examples. Methodologies are discussed briefly as they relate to example applications, and we conclude with a discussion on performance metrics and barriers to implementation.

CURRENT ARTIFICIAL INTELLIGENCE USES AND EXAMPLES
Imaging interpretation/computer vision

Recognition of pathologic condition on imaging is central to surgical practice. Convolution Neural Networks have become a preferred approach in AI image recognition.[1,2] These layered arrays of "neurons," which lead neural networks to be called deep learning, recognize portions of shapes in their lower layers, and compile them into categorizable forms in the upper layers. Published AI applications in medical imaging number in the thousands.[2]

Example: mammography

AI in mammography is part early success and part cautionary tale. Computer-aided detection (CAD), as it came to be called in mammography, was approved by the U.S. Food and Drug Administration (FDA) in 1998 with the ImageChecker system by Hologic (Marlborough, MA).[3,4] Algorithms are trained on images labeled with known pathologic condition[5,6] to assess malignancy risk and to highlight suspicious regions of interest.[6] By 2012, CAD was used in 83% of screening mammograms within the United States National Breast Cancer Surveillance Consortium, as a "second reader" in addition to a radiologist.[7] Medicare began reimbursing for CAD technology in 2002.[5,7]

Although hopes to improve accuracy and decrease human workload were high, studies have been mixed. Some found CAD was associated with increased sensitivity at the expense of decreased specificity and more patient callbacks.[8,9] A 2015 review of greater than 600,000 mammograms found CAD offered no benefit in sensitivity, specificity, or cancer detection rate, and the use of CAD versus human reads was associated with reduced area under the receiver operating characteristic curve (AUROC) for cancer detection from 0.88 to 0.84.[7] Further, radiologists spent time discounting false positives raised by the computer.[5,7]

More recently, the performance of a new CAD system was published by Google Health (Palo Alto, CA), DeepMind (London, UK) and collaborators. Their algorithm, trained on 25,856 UK mammograms and tested on 3097 US mammograms, outperformed radiologists on the test set (9.4% greater sensitivity and 5.7% greater specificity).[10] **Fig. 1** shows example malignancies identified. Notably, UK mammography includes routine double-reading, whereas a single reader is standard in the United States. Thus, it may be partly a better-curated training set that allowed the AI to outperform single US human readers. Although CAD for mammography has been used for several years, its clinical utility has yet to be proven in real-world practice.

Example: portable chest radiograph life-threatening condition detection

AI to identify life-threatening conditions on point-of-care x-rays has the potential to decrease delays in diagnosis and treatment. In 2019, GE Healthcare (General Electric, Boston, MA), in collaboration with researchers University of California San Francisco (UCSF) received FDA 510K clearance for a point-of-care, on-device pneumothorax

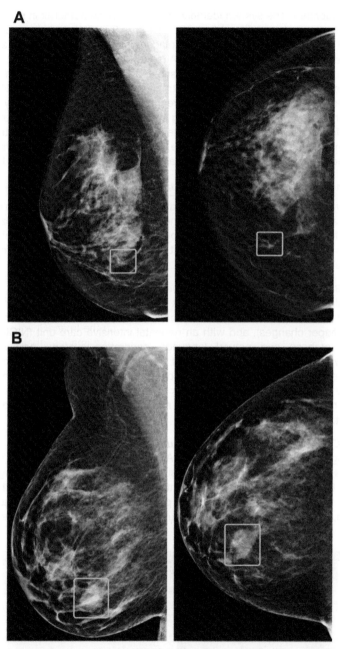

Fig. 1. Discrepancies between the AI system and human readers in 2020 study by McKinney et al. Panel (*A*) highlights a malignancy detected by the AI but missed by human readers. Panel (*B*) shows a malignancy caught by human readers but missed by the AI system. (*From* McKinney SM, Sieniek M, Godbole V, et al. International evaluation of an AI system for breast cancer screening [published correction appears in Nature. 2020 Oct;586(7829):E19]. Nature. 2020;577(7788):89-94; with permission.)

detection algorithm. The system identifies regions of pneumothorax in real time.[11,12] The UCSF team went on to fill out their "Critical Care Suite" of algorithms, developing automated detection of endotracheal tube placement (FDA cleared in 2020) and pneumoperitoneum (**Fig. 2**), which is under FDA review.

The pneumothorax detection algorithm showed a specificity of greater than 95%[12] and has identified pneumothoraces in postmarket testing that were missed by a radiologist. Designed to augment radiologist recognition, the algorithm displays a confidence rating and a heatmap highlighting the region of concern. Transparency is important for building confidence in augmented reads. The algorithm is intended for high-volume centers where reader fatigue is a factor, low resourced environments where a radiologist is not available, and training environments to augment learning.

Text summarization, storytelling, and natural language processing

Health professionals distill complex information into clinical vignettes, which efficiently communicate patient status. When machines lack this ability to contextualize, it fuels our digital frustrations. Programming computers to summarize data into stories, however, holds potential to inform and augment human decision-making and to offload repetitive tasks such as chart review.

Example: BabyTalk for NICU shift summaries
A powerful example is the 2009 BabyTalk project.[13] Neonatal ICU sensor data was processed for events, combined with an annotated timeline of tasks (such as blood draws or diaper changes), and with an neonatal intensive care unit (NICU)-specific ontology database and natural language generation system, processed into machine-written "shift reports." Quality of the reports was assessed by comparing clinician decision quality. Decisions based on the machine-written summaries and graphically presented raw data were comparable but both were inferior to decisions based on human expert summaries. The researchers concluded this to be a proof of concept, with room for growth.

Example: CliniText machine-written care summaries
Functioning on a broader time scale is the AI system CliniText, which wrote discharge summaries following cardiac surgery and summaries of diabetes care during a 5-year interval.[14] Domain knowledge was fed into CliniText, which facilitated the use of abductive reasoning. For example, if a pulmonary artery pressure measurement was found, the algorithm inferred that a pulmonary artery catheter had been placed.

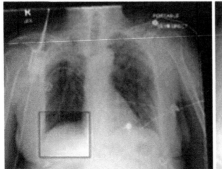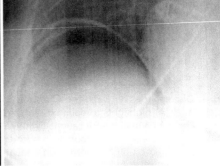

Fig. 2. Heatmap highlighting a region on pneumoperitoneum on chest radiograph; example from the Critical Care Suite of algorithms by UCSF and GE.

On comparison of computer-generated summaries to those written by experts, the algorithm's texts contained a more complete accounting of constituent data but were more likely to lack expert-deemed "important" information.[15]

Example: data-to-text summarization of unstructured data

Neither BabyTalk nor CliniText uses free-text or unstructured data, which is where context and medical reasoning are often found. Scott and colleagues addressed this with their clinical data-to-text system. An AI chart reviewer was developed, which identified events from clinician notes, laboratories and imaging reports, arranged them into a "chronicle" or timeline, then pruned to relevant content, as illustrated in **Fig. 3**.[16–18] Using natural language generation, a textual summary was then constructed.[19] To assess the output, oncology clinicians were given either the full record or the computer's summary and asked to answer questions such as cancer type and prior treatments given. Results showed a slightly higher accuracy (mean 8 vs 7.6 of 10 questions correct) and a remarkable 50% reduction in time to answer the questions when reviewing the summary versus the full record. Clinician response was overwhelmingly positive.[19]

Summarization algorithms may struggle, similar to trainees, to appropriately emphasize key actionable data and deemphasize other information. Studies thus far suggest that processing unstructured text and adding subspecialty domain knowledge both serve to improve the narrative quality.

Trajectory and risk prediction

Prediction of risk and clinical trajectory are central to surgical planning and patient counseling. The uncertainty and multitude of contributing variables make trajectory

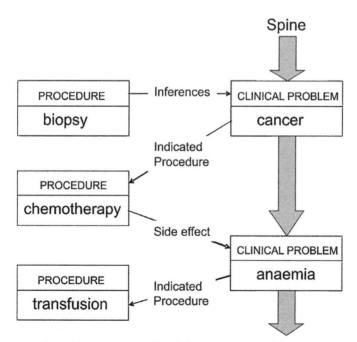

Fig. 3. Content selection by Scott and colleagues' Data-to-Text system, after creation of the comprehensive timeline. (*From* Scott D, Hallett C, Fettiplace R. Data-to-text summarisation of patient records: using computer-generated summaries to access patient histories. Patient Educ Couns. 2013;92(2):153-159. https://doi.org/10.1016/j.pec.2013.04.019.)

prediction a challenging but attractive AI target. Countless disease and field-specific calculators have been developed; we will discuss on several with broad applicability.

Example: National Surgical Quality Improvement Project score

The well-known American College of Surgeons (ACS) Surgical Risk Calculator is a product of the National Surgical Quality Improvement Project (NSQIP), developed in 2013 using data from 1.4 million patients across 393 hospitals. This hierarchical linear regression based model predicts 30-day perioperative morbidity and mortality based on 21 clinical inputs.[20] This was the first calculator designed for use across surgical procedures and patient populations, and revolutionized surgeons' ability to personalize informed consent discussions with patients.[20] Updates to the model with new data continue to be made.[21,22]

Linear regression is familiar to most physicians, and involves assigning relative weights to input variables according to their magnitude of association with an outcome of interest, and summing them to create a prediction. Hierarchical linear regression involves creating multiple linear models that may have different intercepts to reflect nested clustering, for example, hospital level variables, while still elucidating the relationships between lower-level variables such as patient factors.[23,24]

Example: Predictive Optimal Trees in Emergency Surgery Risk score

The ACS NSQIP calculator, similar to any regression model, assumes risk factors interact in linear manner. This is not universally true; for example, a hemoglobin drop from 11 to 9 g/dL is seen differently than a drop from 7 to 5, although they are the same magnitude. The Predictive Optimal Trees in Emergency Surgery Risk (POTTER) calculator, developed in 2020 uses decision trees to address this. The algorithm, trained on 382,960 NSQIP patients undergoing emergency surgery, is visualized as a decision tree with dozens of splits. Risk factors may appear in multiple branches, in varying order, and with differing cutoff values, so traveling various branches of the tree allows factors to interact and "modify" each other's impact on the predicted outcome.[25]

The original decision tree algorithm Classification and Regression Trees (1984), created splits in a top–down manner.[26] Limitations included the need to "prune" the tree after creation to avoid overfitting (matching the dataset so closely that noise is treated as signal), and the problem that, although local patterns might be captured well, larger structures in the data might be missed by chance on suboptimal early split. Multiple tree algorithms have been developed.[27–29] Optimal trees represent a particular answer to decision tree challenges, allowing the algorithm to explore overall dataset structure and split options, before committing to a single "optimal" tree model.[30]

Example: Early Warning Scores

Although forecasting risk preoperatively is useful, expected trajectory evolves over time. The Early Warning Score (EWS) developed in 1997 used physiologic variables to dynamically flag patients at risk for deterioration or cardiac arrest.[31] Updated scores include the Modified Early Warning Score (MEWS)[32] and National Early Warning Score (NEWS).[33,34] Both include temperature, heart rate, systolic blood pressure, respiratory rate, and level of consciousness; NEWS also includes oxygen saturation. These are essentially linear models that use binning to streamline calculation (ie, a systolic blood pressure of 81–100 mmHg yields a blood pressure score of 1 in MEWS[32]), and the total score is summed and mapped to a risk category. MEWS demonstrated AUROC of 0.7 for cardiac arrest or need for ICU,[32] and NEWS yielded AUROC of 0.89 for in-hospital mortality.[33]

Some organizations incorporate EWSs into electronic medical records (EMRs), creating clinician alerts.[35–37] In 2019, for example, the University of Utah's health system reported a 20% decrease in sepsis mortality after implementing MEWS.[37] This showcases that condensing data streams into one signal can help clinicians identify a trend. However, similar to any automated system, MEWS and NEWS suffer from false positives and false negatives. Clinicians may appreciate effective early warnings and loath these scores when they misfire. Triggering of alerts for patients with chronic conditions who are at baseline, or for acute problems already being managed, contributes to provider alarm fatigue.[38,39]

Example: neural network prediction systems

Given the limitations of arithmetical scores such as MEWS, harnessing context, specific to both the patient and medical field, is key to improving predictions. Long short-term memory (LSTM) recurrent neural networks figure prominently in this field[40–43]; they reference information from earlier steps in processing, allowing the past to influence current calculations.[44]

A notable example is Thorson-Meyer and colleagues' work predicting 90-day mortality.[45] They trained an LSTM network on 12,616 intensive care unit (ICU) admissions in Denmark, 42% of which were surgical. Inputs included demographics, diagnoses, laboratories, and vital signs. Their model achieved AUROC of 0.82 on a US validation dataset.[46] Although neural networks are notoriously uninterpretable "black boxes," this team prioritized model interpretability. Using a feature-importance assessment algorithm,[47] infographics, as shown in **Fig. 4**, illustrated which model inputs were driving the result toward survival or nonsurvival over time.

To the authors' knowledge, no neural network trajectory prediction models are in widespread, EMRs-integrated use. There remains uncertainty whether such models will function best as risk assessment tools such as the NSQIP calculator, or as clinician-alert tools such as MEWS/NEWS.

Operative navigation and support

Example: operative navigation in spinal surgery

Minimally invasive surgery requires precise maneuvers through tiny incisions. This is key in positioning of pedicle screws for spinal surgery, where malpositioned screws may cause bleeding, nerve injury, or loss of fixation.[48–50]

In addition to intraoperative imaging, Augmented reality (AR) systems now exist, in which screw path is planned virtually, that is, marking the trajectory on computed tomography (CT) images, and the operator is guided through in vivo placement. The ClarifEye system (Philips, Amsterdam, the Nether-lands)[51] and xvision (Augmedics, Arlington Heights, IL)[52] are examples. Both use intraoperative CT for path planning. Philips' system registers to skin surface fiducials using optical tracking, and Augmedics' system requires marker fixation to bony landmarks. Instrument positions are tracked, and the surgeon sees either on-screen video guidance (Philips), or holographic overlay via an AR headset (Augmedics), to allow matching of the planned screw trajectory. Philips first human study yielded accurate screw placement in 94% of cases, similar to that without AR guidance.[49,51] Augmedics, in its first human study showed 100% accuracy.[52] Although it is unclear whether AR systems substantially improve accuracy in the hands of experts, laboratory models suggest shortened learning curves and improved screw positioning by less experienced operators.[53]

Further, robotic arm systems have also been developed to guide screw placement. After CT and intraoperative registration, a robotic arm is navigated to the planned trajectory, providing a drill guide. The first such system, SpineAssist (Mazor Robotics Inc.,

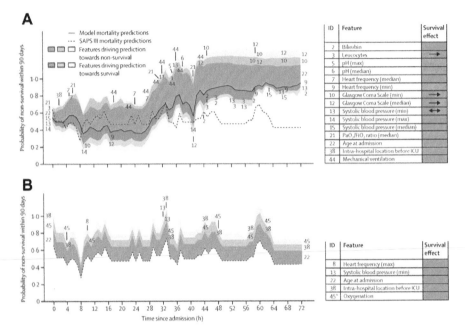

Fig. 4. Infographics showing drivers of AI-predicted survival versus non-survival over time in ICUstudy by Thorson-Meyer et al. The top panel (*A*) shows the model's mortality prediction (solid redline) and the features most driving it towards survival and non-survival at each time point (shaded areas, and key at right). The bottom panel (*B*) shows, for comparison, morality prediction from SAPSIII (Simplified Acute Physiology Score III), and the features most driving its prediction over time. (Reprinted with permission from Elsevier. The Lancet, April 2020, 2 (4), e179–e191.)

Caesarea, Israel) was FDA approved in 2004,[54,55] showing 98% accuracy in screw placement, and decreased fluoroscopy time.[56] Updated platforms continue to be developed.[54] Data suggest a significant reduction in need for reoperation, and approximately 50% reduction in fluoroscopy duration with versus without robot use.[57,58]

Example: surgical robots for soft tissue

The Da Vinci Surgical System (Intuitive, Sunnyvale, CA) became the first FDA-approved laparoscopic robotic platform in 2000. Its wristed instruments, allowing dexterous movements in confined spaces such as the pelvis, contributed to its rapid adoption by urologists. By 2009, the robot was used in 86% of US prostate cancer operations.[59] The Da Vinci system is operated by a human surgeon, seated at a console, with potential enhancements provided by the computer—including magnification, 3D view from the binocular camera and monitor tremor reduction, and in some cases intraoperative alerts.[59,60] Robotic surgery has been criticized for its increased cost relative to laparoscopy[61] and its potential association with loss of laparoscopic skills.[62] Outcome data suggest robot use is associated with decreased short-term pain and blood loss but equivalent long-term and oncologic outcomes.[59,63–65]

An autonomous surgical robot is among the most difficult goals for AI, requiring computer vision, instrument tracking, force sensing, and domain knowledge.[66] These challenges are greater when soft tissue is involved, given its complex deformations.[67] Nevertheless, in 2016 Shademan and colleagues described the Smart Tissue

Anastomosis Robot (STAR), a bowel-sewing robot using near-infrared 3D point tracking of topical indocyanine green markers and mechanical suturing.[68–72] The robot (**Fig. 5**) autonomously planed and placed sutures with appropriate spacing and tension, creating anastomoses in segments of ex vivo porcine bowel, as well as in vivo for 4 live pigs. No leaks were observed on ex vivo pressure testing, or in the pigs, which were sacrificed for examination at 7 days postop. Surgical conditions were highly controlled, with the bowel suspended with stay sutures by a human assistant.[68] Still, the innovations required to build STAR, and its successful functioning on living tissue, suggest a day might come when surgeons work to train robotic modules that will repeat operative steps with efficiency and precision exceeding that of humans.

DISCUSSION

As AI models abound, clinicians must develop literacy in evaluating model development and performance. Attention to quality and representativeness of the training and testing sets is needed, and having an external "validation" set, of data the algorithm has not yet seen, is best practice.

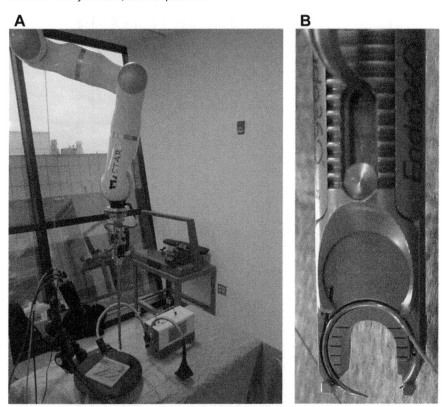

Fig. 5. STAR setup in the laboratory (*A*). The platform uses a modified Endo360° suture device (*B*) (Corporis Medical, Maastricht, the Netherlands). (*From* Leonard S, Wu KL, Kim Y, Krieger A, Kim PC. Smart tissue anastomosis robot (STAR): a vision-guided robotics system for laparoscopic suturing. IEEE Trans Biomed Eng. 2014;61(4):1305-1317. https://doi.org/10.1109/TBME.2014.2302385; with permission.)

Table 1
Common metrics of machine learning model performance

Metric	Meaning	Value in "Perfect" Model	Value in Random Classifier	Accounts for Outcome Prevalence
AUROC (Area under the Receiver Operating Characteristic Curve)	Area under a curve plotting sensitivity (y-axis) vs 1-specificity, that is, false-positive rate (x-axis)	1.0	0.5	No
Sensitivity (Recall)	Given the outcome is present, chance that the model predicts it is present	1.0	0.5	No
Specificity	Given the outcome is absent, chance that the model predicts it is absent	1.0	0.5	No
Positive predictive value (Precision)	Given a positive prediction, chance that the outcome is truly present	1.0	0.5	Yes
Negative predictive value	Given a negative prediction, chance that the outcome is truly absent	1.0	0.5	Yes
C-statistic (Concordance statistical)	Likelihood that a subject experiencing the outcome will have a higher predicted probability of the outcome than a subject who does experience it; evaluates model's ability to rank subjects in order of risk but not its ability to assign absolute probabilities	1.0	0.5	No
Brier Score	Sum of the square of the differences between observed and expected values, divided by the number of observations	0	1.0	Yes
Mean Absolute Error	Sum of the absolute value of the differences between the observed and expected value, divided by the number of observations	0	Varies by quantity predicted	Yes

The "value in random classifier" column assumes a binary classification task, except for Mean Absolute Error, which is generally used for continuous variable prediction.

Regarding model performance, metrics of discrimination (eg, AUROC and c-statistic) describe how correctly a model ranks subjects from more to less likely to experience an outcome.[73,74] Discrimination does not describe how likely a prediction is to be true for any individual; this is described by metrics of calibration, such as the Brier Score or Mean Absolute Error.[75,76] In practice, one must consider the prevalence of the outcome of interest by computing the positive and negative predictive values, which reflect the chance that a positive or negative prediction is true for a given patient. **Table 1** provides definitions of commonly used metrics of model performance. The intended use case must also be considered—for example, if detection is the priority, models with high sensitivity (at the expense of a lower Brier score and higher false-positive rate) may be of greater clinical utility than a model with lower overall error rate.[77]

Although there are many promising systems, AI's growth in health care has been slower than expected for several reasons. First, models are not necessarily transferable from the training setting to a new setting and must be continuously recalibrated. It is only recently that the Minimum Information for Medical AI Reporting standard has been proposed,[78] to facilitate assessment of algorithm applicability across contexts. Further, the predominant business model is selling "final" models to institutions, not suites of tools to evolve algorithms over time. Continuous improvement requires institutions to build data pipelines for secure, continuous reextraction of variables and retraining of algorithms. Yet, due to regulatory and computing infrastructure challenges, data silos are the norm in health care,[79] and few health systems have the personnel, expertise, and budget in place to construct a robust data pipeline for AI.

Further, algorithms learn from the data they see, and will perpetuate the biases of existing systems.[80] For example, Buolawini and colleagues strikingly showed that computer vision algorithms failed to recognize darker-skinned faces as faces, due to gross underrepresentation of dark-skinned individuals in the training sets.[81,82] Both diverse datasets, and adequate labeling and evaluation of model performance with respect to underprivileged groups, are essential to prevent encoding biases into new systems.[79,80]

Finally, no single group has all the information to make AI "work" for health care. Clinicians, data scientists, social scientists, and sharing of data from a range of sources are needed to build AI systems that are relevant, equitable, and dynamic.

SUMMARY

Applications for AI/ML in surgery include image interpretation, data summarization, automated narrative construction, trajectory and risk prediction, operative navigation, and robotics. The pace of AI system development has, overall, exceeded the pace at which such systems can be validated, assessed for clinical utility and equity, and deployed into clinical practice. Some AI tools are already in operation and working well but adequate data infrastructure and novel multidisciplinary teams will be needed to grow AI into an every-day asset for surgeons.

CLINICS CARE POINTS

- Numerous predictive algorithms, for diagnosis and prognosis, exist in the literature. Key considerations before applying an algorithm to a patient's condition include whether the algorithm wastrained on a population similar to one's own patients, and whether the algorithm has a meansfor continuous updating over time.

- The performance of classification algorithms is often reported in terms of area under the receiver operating characteristic curve (AUROC). AUROC describes, in one number, how a model performs across a range of possible decision thresholds. To place this number in context, it isadvisable for clinicians to also choose a sensitivity (or specificity) threshold, and to calculatethe positive (or negative) predictive value based on the condition's prevalence in their patientpopulation. This will allow clinicians to answer the question, "Given a positive prediction fromthe algorithm, how likely is the outcome to actually occur?"

- Machine learning algorithms have often been described as interpretable or uninterpretable ("blackbox"). Interpretable methods, such as linear and logistic regression and single decision treemodels, may provide numerical weights or decision thresholds for humans to follow how theiroutput is arrived at. Less interpretable methods may include neural networks and ensemblemodels (i.e. Random Forest, which sums the results of numerous decision trees). One typeis not routinely better than the other, and advances like post-hoc explainability algorithmsand highlighting of regions of interest are helping to make previously opaque methods moretransparent.

- The options for applying artificial intelligence and machine learning in-line with clinical practice are growing. Expansion of data infrastructure and input from both clinicians and informaticists/data scientists will be needed to support this continued growth.

DISCLOSURE

Intellectual property for the development of GE Healthcare's Critical Care Suite of algorithms is owned by the University of California and licensed to GE Healthcare. University of California receives royalties from GE, and Dr R. Callcut as an investigator receives a portion. The other authors have nothing to disclose.

REFERENCES

1. Esteva A, Chou K, Yeung S, et al. Deep learning-enabled medical computer vision. NPJ Digit Med 2021;4:1–9. Number: 1 Publisher: Nature Publishing Group.
2. Litjens G, Kooi T, Bejnordi Babak E, et al. A survey on deep learning in medical image analysis. Med Image Anal 2017;42:60–88.
3. Mat Isa Nor Ashidi, Amylia Harsa, Mat Sakim Harsa. Computer-Aided Detection and Diagnosis for Microcalcifications in Mammogram: A Review 2022.
4. Hologic . ImageChecker® 2D CAD Technology 2022.
5. Kohli A, Jha S. Why CAD failed in mammography. J Am Coll Radiol 2018;15: 535–7. Publisher: Elsevier.
6. Oyelade Olaide Nathaniel, Ezugwu Absalom El-Shamir. A state-of-the-art survey on deep learn- ing methods for detection of architectural distortion from digital mammography. IEEE Access 2020;8:148644–76. Conference Name: IEEE Access.
7. Lehman Constance D, Wellman Robert D, Buist Diana SM, et al. Diagnostic accuracy of digital screening mammography with and without computer-aided detection. JAMA Intern Med 2015;175:1828–37.
8. Nishikawa RM, Schmidt RA, Linver MN, et al. Clinically missed cancer: how effectively can radiologists use computer-aided detection? Am J Roentgenol 2012; 198:708–16.
9. Fenton Joshua J, Abraham Linn, Taplin Stephen H, et al. Effectiveness of computer-aided detection in community mammography practice. JNCI: J Natl Cancer Inst 2011;103:1152–61.

10. McKinney SM, Sieniek M, Godbole V, et al. International evaluation of an AI system for breast cancer screening *Nature*, 577, 2020. p. 89–94. Number: 7788 Publisher: Nature Publishing Group.
11. Bai Nina. Artificial Intelligence That Reads Chest X-Rays Is Approved by FDA UC San Francisco 2019.
12. Healthcare GE. Critical care suite on mobile and fixed x-ray systems. GE Healthcare; 2022.
13. Portet F, Reiter E, Gatt A, et al. Automatic generation of textual summaries from neonatal intensive care data. Artif Intelligence 2009;173:789–816.
14. Goldstein A, Shahar Y. Generation of natural-language textual summaries from lon- gitudinal clinical records MEDINFO 2015. eHealth-enabled health 2015;594–8. IOS Press.
15. Goldstein A, Shahar Y. An automated knowledge-based textual summarization system for longitudinal, multivariate clinical data. J Biomed Inform 2016;61: 159–75.
16. Hallett Catalina, Scott Donia. Structural variation in generated health reports in Proceedings of the Third International Workshop on Paraphrasing (IWP2005) 2005.
17. Hallett C, Power R, Scott D. Summarisation and visualisation of e-Health data repositories in Proceedings of the UK e-science all hands meeting 2006.
18. Harkema Henk, Roberts Ian, Gaizauskas Robert, et al. Information Extraction from Clinical Records in Proceedings of the UK e-Science All Hands Meeting 2005.
19. Scott D, Hallett C, Fettiplace R. Data-to-text summarisation of patient records: Using computer-generated summaries to access patient histories. Patient Educ Couns 2013;92:153–9.
20. Bilimoria Karl Y, Liu Y, Paruch Jennifer L, et al. Development and Evaluation of the Universal ACS NSQIP Surgical Risk Calculator: A Decision Aid and Informed Consent Tool for Patients and Surgeons. J Am Coll Surg 2013;217:833–42.e3.
21. Liu Yaoming, Cohen Mark E, Hall Bruce L, et al. Evaluation and Enhancement of Calibration in the American College of Surgeons NSQIP Surgical Risk Calculator. J Am Coll Surg 2016;223:231–9.
22. Hornor Melissa A, Ma Meixi, Zhou Lynn, et al. Enhancing the American College of Surgeons NSQIP Surgical Risk Calculator to Predict Geriatric Outcomes. J Am Coll Surg 2020;230:88–100.e1.
23. Woltman H, Feldstain A, MacKay J, et al. An Introduction to Hierarchical Lin- ear Modeling. Tutorials in Quantitative Methods for Psychology, 8, 52-69. Quantitative Methods Psychol tutorial 2012;8:52–69.
24. Cohen Mark E, Ko Clifford Y, Bilimoria Karl Y, et al. Optimizing ACS NSQIP modeling for eval- uation of surgical quality and risk: patient risk adjustment, procedure mix adjustment, shrinkage adjustment, and surgical focus. J Am Coll Surg 2013;217:336–46.e1.
25. Bertsimas D, Dunn J, Velmahos George C, et al. Surgical Risk is not linear: derivation and validation of a novel, user-friendly, and machine-learning-based predictive optimal trees in emergency surgery risk (POTTER) Calculator. Ann Surg 2018;268:574–83.
26. Breiman L, Friedman Jerome H, Olshen Richard A, et al. Classification and Regression trees. Boca Raton, Fla: Chapman and Hall/CRC1st edition; 1984.
27. Breiman Leo. Random Forests. Machine Learn 2001;45:5–32.
28. Kingsford C, Salzberg SL. What are decision trees? Nat Biotechnol 2008;26: 1011–3. Number: 9 Publisher: Nature Publishing Group.

29. Chen T, Guestrin C. XGBoost: a scalable tree boosting system Proceedings of the 22nd ACM SIGKDD international Conference on knowledge Discovery and data mining. arXiv 2016;785–794. 1603.02754.

30. Bertsimas Dimitris, Dunn Jack. Optimal classification trees. Machine Learn 2017; 106:1039–82.

31. Morgan RJM, William F, Wright MM. An early warning scoring system for detecting developing critical. Illness 1997;8:100.

32. Subbe CP, Kruger M, Rutherford P, et al. Validation of a modified Early Warning Score in medical admissions. QJM: monthly J Assoc Physicians 2001;94:521–6.

33. Royal College of Physicians of London. National early warning score (NEWS): standardising the assessment of acute-illness severity in the NHS. London, UK: Royal College of Physicians; 2012. OCLC, 810424414.

34. Physicians Royal College. National Early Warning Score (NEWS2) standardising the assessment of acute-illness severity in the NHS (London). London, UK: Royal College of Physicians; 2017.

35. Shelley Schoepflin Sanders Scott Marsal. An electronic modified early warning system can reduce mortality. Harv Business Rev 2013. Section: Health and behavioral science.

36. UK Cerner. Keeping the nurse at the bedside: implementing electronic recording of the national early warning score. United Kingdom: Cerner; 2015.

37. Siwicki B. Health system uses Epic EHR, communications tech to reduce sepsis mortality rate by 20%. Healthcare IT News 2019.

38. Eccles Sinan R, Subbe C, Hancock D, et al. improving speci- ficity whilst maintaining sensitivity of the National Early Warning Score in patients with chronic hypoxaemia. Resuscitation 2014;85:109–11.

39. Keim-Malpass J, Clark Matthew T, Lake Douglas E, Moorman JR. Towards development of alert thresholds for clinical deterioration using continuous predictive analytics mon- itoring. J Clin Monit Comput 2020;34:797–804.

40. Shickel B, Tighe Patrick J, Bihorac A, Rashidi P. Deep EHR: a survey of recent advances in deep learning techniques for electronic health record (EHR) analysis. IEEE J Biomed Health Inform 2018;22:1589–604. Conference Name: IEEE Journal of Biomedical and Health Informatics.

41. Guo Aixia, Beheshti R, Khan Yosef M, et al. Pre- dicting cardiovascular health trajectories in time-series electronic health records with LSTM mod- els. BMC Med Inform Decis Mak 2021;21:5.

42. Saqib M, Sha Y, Wang May D. Early prediction of sepsis in EMR records using traditional ML Techniques and Deep Learning LSTM Networks in 2018. EMBC 2018;4038–4041:1558–4615.

43. Yin C, Zhao R, Qian B, et al. Domain knowledge guided deep learning with electronic health records in *2019*. IEEE international Conference on data mining (ICDM) 2019;738–747:2374–8486.

44. Staudemeyer Ralf C, Morris Eric R. Understanding LSTM – a tutorial into long short- term memory recurrent neural networks. arXiv 2019;1909:09586 [cs].

45. Thorsen-Meyer HC, Nielsen Annelaura B, Nielsen Anna P, et al. Dynamic and explainable machine learning prediction of mortality in patients in the intensive care unit: a ret- rospective study of high-frequency data in electronic patient records. Lancet Digital Health 2020;2:e179–91.

46. Johnson Alistair EW, Pollard Tom J, Shen L, et al. MIMIC-III, a freely accessible critical care database. Sci Data 2016;3:160035. Number: 1 Publisher: Nature Publishing Group.

47. Lundberg S, Lee S. In. A Unified Approach to Interpreting Model Predictions. arXiv 2017;1705:07874, cs, stat].

48. Tian NF, Huang QS, Zhou P, et al. Pedicle screw insertion accuracy with different assisted methods: a systematic review and meta-analysis of comparative studies. Eur Spine J 2011;20:846–59.

49. Gelalis Ioannis D, Paschos Nikolaos K, Pakos Emilios E, et al. Accuracy of pedicle screw place- ment: a systematic review of prospective in vivo studies comparing free hand, fluoroscopy guidance and navigation techniques. Eur Spine J 2012;21:247–55.

50. Tang J, Zhu Z, Sui T, et al. Position and complications of pedicle screw insertion with or without image-navigation techniques in the thoracolumbar spine: a meta-analysis of comparative studies. J Biomed Res 2014;28:228–39.

51. Elmi-Terander A, Burström G, Nachabe R, et al. Pedicle screw placement using augmented reality surgical navigation with intraoperative 3d imaging: a first in-human prospective cohort study. Spine 2019;44:517–25.

52. Yahanda Alexander T, Moore E, Ray Wilson Z, et al. First in-human report of the clinical accuracy of thoracolumbar percutaneous pedicle screw placement using augmented reality guidance. Neurosurg Focus 2021;51:E10. Publisher: American Association of Neurological Surgeons Section: Neurosurgical Focus.

53. Dennler C, Jaberg L, Spirig J, et al. Augmented reality-based navigation increases precision of pedicle screw insertion. J Orthopaedic Surg Res 2020; 15:174.

54. Vadal'a G, Salvatore SD, Ambrosio L, et al. Robotic spine surgery and augmented reality systems: a state of the art. Neurospine 2020;17:88–100.

55. Dreval' ON, Rynkov IP, Kasparova KA, et al. [Results of using Spine Assist Mazor in surgical treatment of spine disorders]. Zh Vopr Neirokhir Im N N Burdenko 2014;78:14–20.

56. Dijk Joris D, Ende Roy PJ, Stramigioli S, et al. Clinical pedicle screw accuracy and deviation from planning in robot-guided spine surgery: robot-guided pedicle screw accuracy. Spine 2015;40:E986–91.

57. Kantelhardt SR, Martinez R, Baerwinkel S, Burger R, et al. Perioperative course and accuracy of screw positioning in conventional, open robotic-guided and percutaneous robotic-guided, pedicle screw placement. Eur Spine J 2011;20: 860–8.

58. Fan Y, Du J, Zhang J, et al. Comparison of accuracy of pedicle screw insertion among 4 guided technologies in spine surgery. Med Sci Monit 2017;23:5960–8.

59. Bec Crew. Worth the cost? A closer look at the da Vinci robot's impact on prostate cancer surgery. Nature 2020;580:S5–7. Bandiera abtest: a Cg type: Nature Index Number: 7804 Publisher: Nature Publishing Group Subject term: Cancer, Engineering, Industry.

60. Song Hyunwoo, Moradi Hamid, Jiang Baichuan, et al. Real-time intraoperative surgical guidance system in the da Vinci surgical robot based on transrectal ultrasound/photoacoustic imaging with photoacoustic markers: an ex vivo demonstration 2022.

61. Boggs Will. Robotic-assisted surgery: more expensive, but not always more effective Reuters.2017.

62. Abaza R. The robotic surgery era and the role of laparoscopy training. Ther Adv Urol 2009;1:161–5.

63. Coughlin Geoffrey D, Yaxley John W, Chambers Suzanne K, et al. Robot-assisted laparoscopic prostatectomy versus open radical retropubic prostatectomy: 24-

month outcomes from a ran- domised controlled study. Lancet Oncol 2018;19: 1051–60.

64. Zhou JY, Xin C, Mou YP, et al. Robotic versus laparoscopic distal pancreatectomy: a meta-analysis of short-term outcomes. PLoS One 2016;11:e0151189. Publisher: Public Library of Science.

65. Baik Seung H, Kwon HY, Kim Jin S, et al. Robotic versus laparoscopic low anterior resection of rectal cancer: short-term outcome of a prospective comparative study. Ann Surg Oncol 2009;16:1480–7.

66. Panesar S, Cagle Y, Chander D, et al. Artificial intelligence and the future of surgical robotics. Ann Surg 2019;270:223–6.

67. Golse N, Petit A, Lewin M, et al. Augmented reality during open liver surgery using a markerless non-rigid registration system. J Gas- trointestinal Surg 2021;25: 662–71.

68. Shademan A, Decker Ryan S, Opfermann Justin D, et al. Supervised autonomous robotic soft tissue surgery. Sci Transl Med 2016;8:337ra64. American Association for the Advancement of Science.

69. Shademan A, Dumont Matthieu F, Leonard S, et al. Feasi- bility of near-infrared markers for guiding surgical robots in. Opt Model Perform Predictions VI 2013; 8840:123–32.

70. Leonard S, Shademan A, Kim Y, et al. Smart Tissue Anas- tomosis Robot (STAR): Accuracy evaluation for supervisory suturing using near-infrared fluores- cent markers in 2014. IEEE international Conference on Robotics and automation (ICRA) 2014;1889–1894:1050–4729.

71. Leonard S, Wu Kyle L, Kim Y, et al. Smart tissue anasto- mosis robot (STAR): a vision-guided robotics system for laparoscopic suturing. IEEE Trans Actions Biomed Eng 2014;61:1305–17. Conference Name: IEEE Transactions on Biomedical Engineering.

72. Decker R, Shademan A, Opfermann J, et al. Performance evaluation and clinical applications of 3D plenoptic cameras in next-generation robotics machine intelligence bio-inspired. Comput Theor Appl IX 2015;9494:62–72.

73. Hanley JA, McNeil BJ. The meaning and use of the area under a receiver operating charac- teristic (ROC) curve. Radiology 1982;143:29–36.

74. Pencina Michael J, D'Agostino Ralph B. Evaluating discrimination of risk prediction models: the C statistic. JAMA 2015;314:1063–4.

75. Fenlon C, O'Grady L, Doherty ML, et al. A discussion of calibra- tion techniques for evaluating binary and categorical predictive models. Prev Vet Med 2018;149: 107–14.

76. Huang Y, Li W, Macheret F, et al. A tu- torial on calibration measurements and calibration models for clinical prediction models. J Am Med Inform Assoc 2020;27: 621–33.

77. Assel Melissa, Sjoberg Daniel D, Vickers Andrew J. The Brier score does not evaluate the clinical utility of diagnostic tests or prediction models. Diagn Progn Res 2017;1:1–7. Number: 1 Publisher: BioMed Central.

78. Hernandez-Boussard T, Bozkurt S, Ioannidis John PA, Shah Nigam H. MINIMAR (MIN- imum Information for Medical AI Reporting): developing reporting standards for artificial intelli- gence in health care. J Am Med Inform Assoc 2020; 27:2011–5. Publisher: Oxford Academic.

79. Lam Kyle, Abramoff Michael D, Balibrea José M, et al. A Delphi consensus statement for digital surgery. NPJ Dig Med 2022;5:1–9. Number: 1 Publisher: Nature Publishing Group.

80. O'Reilly-Shah Vikas N, Gentry Katherine R, Walters Andrew M, et al. Bias and ethical considerations in machine learning and the automation of perioperative risk assessment. BJA: Br J Anaesth 2020;125:843–6.
81. Buolamwini J, Gebru T. Gender shades: Intersectional accuracy disparities in commercial gender classification. Conf Fairness, Account Transparency 2018; 81:77–91.
82. Creative Commons — Attribution 4.0 International — CC BY 4.0.

Beyond the Spreadsheet
Data Management for Physicians in the Era of Big Data

Carly Eckert, MD, MPH

KEYWORDS

• Data management • Data governance • Big Data • Databases

KEY POINTS

- Big Data management requires new and advanced skills and tools.
- Physician familiarity with the Big Data management lifecycle is crucial to be efficient and productive researchers.
- Physician collaboration with information technology professionals can facilitate Big Data analytics and applications.

INTRODUCTION

Physicians are well-versed in the explosion of data that have impacted their lives and livelihoods. They have learned about Big Data, the internet of things, and the vaunted promise of precision medicine. However, despite familiarity with these phrasings, few have a background or formal training in Big Data management. Although spreadsheets may have served their research and exploratory data analysis requirements a decade ago, these tools now fall short of the demands of Big Data. Indeed, one of the characteristics of Big Data is that traditional methods of data management and analysis are insufficient. So how do physicians level up their skills and understanding to formulate and answer the questions they have in their practices, operating rooms, and research labs? How do they remain good partners to biostatisticians, data scientists, and information technology (IT) teams to facilitate research and grant applications? The fundamentals and vernacular of Big Data management can serve surgeon scientists well and keep them in the essential conversations of determining how best to use data, including how to interpret the findings and their applications to benefit their practices and patients.

Department of Epidemiology, University of Washington, 1023 Cleland Drive, Chapel Hill, NC 27517, USA
E-mail address: carly.m.eckert@gmail.com
Twitter: @md-carly (C.E.)

Surg Clin N Am 103 (2023) 335–346
https://doi.org/10.1016/j.suc.2022.11.007
0039-6109/23/© 2022 Elsevier Inc. All rights reserved.

Basics of Big Data in Health Care

Big Data results from computing advances that have allowed data to be collected, stored, and analyzed more cheaply and efficiently than ever before. These computing advances have affected health care, as they have affected every industry. These advances have digitized data within and across health systems and given technology professionals and physicians new tools to store, access, and analyze this data.[1] Big Data in health care is characterized by the 5 "V"s: volume, velocity, variety, veracity, and value.[1,2]

1. *Volume.* The quantity of data generated, collected, and available for analysis and use. Based on current estimates, the health care industry generates approximately 30% of the world's data.[3]
2. *Velocity.* The speed at which data are generated and collected. Velocity can include the quasi-instantaneous data generation from patient-centric streaming devices and the nightly loads that transfer structured data to databases from source systems. Furthermore, data consumers increasingly expect data to be rapidly managed, analyzed, and accessible for use.[1]
3. *Variety.* The multitude of sources that contribute to the health care data ecosystem. The variety includes data from the electronic medical record (EMR) and data generated across diverse source systems, including administrative, billing, surgical scheduling, employee, pharmacy, device and supply chain, and machine data from sensors and instruments.[4] Although there is variety within the types of source systems contributing to the data store, there is also variety among the types of data generated by these sources. There are three categories of data types:
   - *Structured data.* Data that are stored as discrete data points such as fields within an electronic health record like "age," "gender," and "diagnosis." Structured data are parsed easily by computers and easily queried by humans.
   - *Unstructured data:* Information stored in aggregate, such as the narrative portion of a clinical note. Unstructured data include medical images, videos, audio, and other file types. These data type can be discretized via natural language processing.[5]
   - *Semi-structured data:* Data whose structure includes organizational features such as tags that allow search capabilities but without the defined domains of structured data.
4. *Veracity.* The ability of the data to capture the truth or the accuracy of the data. This data characteristic is unique to health care data and relates to the expectation that the data generated and collected is error free and credible.[1]
5. *Value:* the usefulness of the data to inform decisions or aid discovery in health care.

Data must be useable, useful, and used to impact health care systems. The remainder of this article highlights the people, processes, and technology involved in transforming data into information, of which the physicians reading this article are an integral part.

Introduction to Data Management

Data management encompasses the lifecycle of data in an organization from the time of data collection until end users consume the data. As we introduce terms and concepts that are integral to the management, use, and application of Big Data, we will use the framework of the data management lifecycle. Although there is some variation in the included components in the data management lifecycle, general elements follow.[6]

Data generation
Data are generated throughout patient care, administrative processes, and facility operations.

For example, hospital staff and employees generate data related to call schedules, shift assignments, and pay calendars. In addition, data are generated by pharmaceutical systems (such as a Pyxis machine) and supply chain systems. Operating rooms generate data for each procedure conducted. Radiology departments generate data from CT scans, MRIs, and other imaging forms. Medical device data, including electrocardiograms and vital sign monitors, generate data, often continuously. Furthermore, wearable devices, such as Holter monitors, defibrillators, and fitness trackers, generate data that health systems may store and analyze.

Data collection
Source systems, such as EMRs, collect data from patient encounters and administrative processes in various ways—including direct data entry, billing transactions, and others.[4] These source systems are systems of record and are updated in near realtime as clinical and business processes occur. In addition, source systems extract data identified by the health system as necessary or desired for operations and analytics at predetermined intervals.[7] Data extracted from source systems is the initial component of a process called "ETL" or "extract–transform–load." ETL processes refer to the three critical stages involved in data movement across systems, processes owned by data engineers.[8] Steps 3 and 4 of this section describe ETL's transform and load stages.

- *Enterprise data warehouse (EDW).* A centralized data repository to which data are extracted regularly from source systems. Data warehouses have a significant level of internal organizing structure that supports functions such as indexing, cataloging, and locating data records.[8] The EDW can be a source for internal reporting and analytics, a substrate for data marts for specific data processes, or a place to pull data for specific analytic questions or research.[7] The data elements pulled and updated from the hospital's source systems can be scoped according to their needs to facilitate business intelligence and reporting needs.[4] Data pipelines connect source systems to EDWs, enabling data to be continually pulled and updated per the predefined cadence.[9]

Data in Context

As data are collected, it is critical to document the context of the data, including the data's original intended use, to provide users and consumers of data applications assurance of its accuracy and validity.[10] Documenting the original context under which the data was collected is also critical for the reproducibility of research and analyses, transparency, and auditability.[11] This context can include the specification of an exam (eg, fasting blood glucose in pregnancy) or the larger social context of a trend (eg, surgical case patterns during 2020).

- *Metadata.* Data about the data. Metadata includes information about the content and organization of data within the database and details on how to access data across different parameters.[12]
- *Data dictionary.* A table within a data store that includes details about each data table and the attributes within each table. A data dictionary explicitly defines included features. The data dictionary should also have a detailed description of each feature. Many data dictionaries will have additional information, such as the data type of the attribute (eg, integer, categorical, or binary) and the

allowed range of values for each attribute, also known as its domain. In addition, the data dictionary includes a key for categorical variables translating each category to its meaning. Data dictionaries also have information about data missingness, a common finding in health care data. Data may be missing for many reasons, including data entry error, a null result, or an attribute irrelevant to a specific encounter (eg, "the absence of medical events are not recorded in health care data sets"). Many databases will use indicators such as 9, -1, n/a, or a blank field to indicate a specific type of missingness that the data dictionary should explain.

- *Data provenance.* A type of metadata that describes the environment in which the data were generated and collected. Data provenance may include details about the data's source systems, such as version number and the time and date the data extract occurred as well as the original intended use of collected data.[10]

Data processing

The data processing needs of Big Data, particularly that of health care Big Data, is one factor that necessitates more advanced tooling and expertise in this field. As described, several characteristics make Big Data challenging to manage. These challenges are magnified when such data must be processed and queried promptly. Once the data have been extracted from the source system and loaded into the EDW or data mart, personnel and automated routines must process it to prepare it for analytics, research, and reporting.

- *Data wrangling or data munging.* Health care data are criticized as messy or noisy. Unfortunately, most real-world data have some degree of noise. Therefore, evaluating and reducing the noise is essential to maximize the data's utility in downstream applications. Data engineers or data scientists must first preprocess the data to prepare it for downstream use, a time-consuming task. Preprocessing can include data validation checks to assess data quality, data normalization, imputation (if appropriate), filtering or cohorting of data, and removal of outliers or nonsensical values.[13,14] Data transformations, augmentation, and enrichment may also occur during this step leading to novel feature generation (eg, computing a new variable as BMI from existing height and weight variables). For data scientists, preprocessing can be inglorious work, occupying 80% of their time.
- *Ontologies and terminologies.* Health standards organizations formulated medical terminologies and ontologies decades ago to standardize billing and administrative processes within and across health institutions. Terminologies such as ICD-10 (International Classification of Diseases, 10th Revision) and CPT (Current Procedural Terminology) codes are common structured data elements stored in data warehouses for data consumers such as data scientists, analysts, and researchers. These terminologies and their varying levels of granularity can be helpful for data scientists to understand and employ for added value during this stage of data management. For example, there are nearly 70,000 ICD-10 CM codes. Many of these codes occur sparsely in care settings and including all of them in analytics projects or predictive modeling would be overwhelming. Preprocessing these codes, and working with subject matter experts such as physicians, can intelligently reduce the number of codes included or "roll them up" to a less granular level, thereby decreasing the feature space.
- *Common data models.* Besides terminologies, health care data can be mapped to common data models (CDMs). CDMs address health care's long challenges with data conformity and interoperability. Although the widespread adoption of

EMRs has spurred data digitization, it has yet to promote data conformity across institutions. EMR vendors have different data schemas and models, making data exchange challenging, if not prohibitive.[15] In part 11 of this collection Drs. Abid and Schneider explain the EMR-associated challenges related to interoperability and data conformity. CDMs can facilitate multi-organizational research and cross-institutional data collaborations as they map data to common formats.[16,17] Interoperability initiatives were initially pioneered in the 1980s for inter-system data conformity and have gained traction to enable semantic interoperability across health systems, although usually catering to the unique needs of a project or initiative. Although many CDMs exist, a few worth noting include:

○ The Observational Medical Outcomes Partnership (OMOP),
○ PCORnet common data model (PCORnet CDM),
○ Informatics for Integrating Biology and the Bedside (i2b2).[17]

Finally, Health Level 7 (HL7), the health data standards organization, manages Fast Healthcare Interoperability Resources (FHIR). FHIR is a data standard that includes the technology to share data across institutions (via APIs, the exact mechanism other wireless transactions use) and the data model based on existing medical terminologies.[18]

- *Data validation.* Sometimes considered one of the steps in the data wrangling process, data validation includes assessing if the data are fit for use.[19] Data validation is a component of data processing that benefits from cross-disciplinary collaboration. Clinicians, business users, or subject domain experts should be involved to validate the data and to ensure that the data are processed in such a way that will answer the research question. For example, if the team is building a model to predict the length of stay following admission to the hospital, is the dataset filtered to only include inpatient admissions? Overlooking the importance of multidisciplinary collaboration during this component of data management could reduce the process's efficiency by requiring rework, or, even worse, generating a faulty result based on data that need to be validated as appropriate for the business need.[20]

Data storage

Storing vast amounts of diverse and heterogenous health care data is a challenging task. Health systems employ large teams of specialized professionals whose whole responsibility is to ensure that data are extracted, stored, and loaded in a way that provides security, compliance, and data use expectations. These teams work to manage terabytes of data while coordinating tooling and products across various vendors with complex scheduled tasks across the landscape of source systems and servers. This section will provide basic definitions of different types of data storage used within health systems. Note that the simplicity of these definitions belies tremendous, cross-functional enterprise-wide efforts that are often very expensive and human-intensive for institutions to do and to do well.[7,9]

- *Database.* A storage location for a collection of data, can range in size from a single flat file to many petabytes.
- *Database management system:* an organized way of collecting and storing data enabling end users to query and analyze data.
- *Enterprise data* warehouse *(EDW).* A centralized and stable data repository designed to host data that is of significant business interest to a health system.[4] Database architects build and maintain the EDW with functions that support queries, analyses, and report generation. EDWs are centralized databases that

are often slow to adapt to changes in data needs and are not built for specialized queries or functions.[4] Most EDWs are relational databases and are performant with structured data elements.

- *Data mart.* A subsection of a data warehouse that is built specifically for a particular business function or a group of business users; an EDW can be composed of multiple data marts.
- *Clinical data* repository. A patient-centric database formed from integrating multiple databases within a health system that allows immediate access to data for research or business use cases. Clinical Data Repositories may contain personally identifiable information, depending on the use case and security requirements.[4,8,21]
- *Data lake.* A large repository for data of any type (including unstructured and semi-structured data) in which data exist in its raw form. Data lakes are less structured than data warehouses and therefore have the advantage of increased flexibility. However, this increased flexibility is tempered by requiring additional effort to use the data by imposing a schema at that time.[22,23]

Types of Databases

Relational databases. Data maintained within tables with a predefined structure and schema. Tables consist of rows and columns. Rows contain the instances: the data about a patient, an encounter, a procedure, or a laboratory event. Columns contain the variables or features, those structured data elements that characterize the instance maintained in the rows. The cell is the intersection of a row and a column and contains a discrete data element, such as the heart rate of a specific patient during one encounter. Relational databases contain structured data and may be as simple as a few flat files linked by a unique identifier to many files requiring complex joins to access and use.

Relational databases rely on a data schema to enforce the database's organizing principles. A data schema is the relationship of the data elements to each other. As the number of tables multiplies and the joins between them become complex, a schema can help the users better understand how to use and generate appropriate queries for the data and schema. Although relational databases are relatively easy to query, there are challenges in scaling and accommodating unstructured or semi-structured data types with relational databases.[24]

- *Relational database management systems (RDBMS).* The software that data consumers use to access data within a relational database. Usually, RDBMS support direct query and application use. This software has several objectives[25]:
  - *Data availability.* Data available to appropriate users in a useable format facilitating access
  - *Data integrity.* The data available are correct and reliable
  - *Data security.* Access control permissions are enforced, limiting use to appropriate users
  - *Data independence.* It allows users to store, query, and update data without concern for the underlying data storage and representation.
- *Unique subject identification number* An alphanumeric identifier assigned to a particular entry (row) in a database; this identifier has no meaning outside of the database and serves to "de-link" data from the personal identifiers to maintain study security and patient data privacy.[24]
- *Primary key.* The variable (or column) that links one table to another. For example, in a database of surgical cases, the case log file may include a column "case ID."

This column links to other tables containing the same column, such as a table mapping case IDs to patient IDs and a table mapping case IDs to the primary surgeon.
- *Foreign key.* Another column or variable that relates one table to another. For example, a surgical case log may have a column that lists the CPT code associated with each case. That CPT code is a foreign key that relates to the CPT code table where each CPT code is mapped to its description.[24]
- *Schema.* A machine-readable definition of the organization of a database.[12]
- *SQL:* Structured Query Language. The programming language, pronounced "see-quel," used to access and query relational data management systems.

NoSQL. It stands for "not only SQL." NoSQL (pronounced No-sequel) databases are an alternative to relational databases. NoSQL databases allow more flexibility in the data they can represent (for example, documents and other non-structured data types) and in their schemas (some can be schema-less!).[26] NoSQL databases can also scale quickly and work well in distributed computing environments. NoSQL databases include key-value stores, document stores, column-oriented databases, and graph databases.[26] However, NoSQL databases require more advanced tooling to access, query, and use the data, limiting the user base. In addition, NoSQL databases tend to be open-source tools with fewer security controls and rigor than relational databases.

Data governance
Data governance is a necessary framework for establishing practices around data access, monitoring, and data use evaluation. Much of this will be standard practice for surgeon researchers due to familiarity with Human Subjects Research training and Institutional Review Board policies and requirements. For a thorough overview of US privacy law and the Health Information Portability and Accountability Act (HIPAA), please see Part 11 of this collection.

Additional data governance concepts related to Big Data management include:

- *Access controls and data use permissions.* In a health system, hundreds of people may need and or want access to data sources for queries or analytics. Data permission procedures must be in place to delegate access to different data systems and to monitor who is accessing the data and when. Such access controls are essential for audit purposes and in cases of data breaches.
  - RBAC. Role-based access control. Permission to access various data systems and servers is based on the user's role. The permissions allow access to specific components or elements of databases or servers per the role requirements.[12]
  - ABAC. Attribute-based access control. Attributes associated with the user, the system, or the environment define the permitting of access.
- *Secondary data use.* One of the purposes of Big Data management is to facilitate the appropriate use of collected data for the health system's business, operational, and care needs. For data to be reusable, the proposed use cases must align with the institution's governance and data stewardship procedures.[27] Secondary use policies may dictate, for example, that only deidentified data are available for reuse within the health system. Alternatively, specialized research data marts may be instantiated that provide identifiable health information for IRB-approved purposes.[4]
- *Metadata management.* As mentioned earlier in this article, metadata is crucial to understanding data as it provides the necessary context. Data governance policies manage systems metadata which includes data lineage.

○ *Data* lineage. A record of the steps, processes, and procedures that occurred to the data from the time it was generated to the time it is used, including how data were processed and potentially altered from its original state.[28]

Data analysis

Data become information as these become organized and capable of driving decisions or discovery.[12] The prior stages of the data management lifecycle serve to collect and organize data and prepare it for subsequent analysis. This analysis stage may include regular reports from data analysts for departmental review or business intelligence tools that allow nontechnical user interaction. Data analysis also includes work by data scientists to mine large databases to find novel patterns that may provide new insights into care processes or system operations. As discussed, Big Data analyses require more than traditional analytical tools. In other industries, Big Data platforms, cloud computing, and data virtualization are all commonly used to analyze Big Data adequately and efficiently. Using these tools in health care environments can be challenging given the skill sets required, the open-source nature of these platforms, and the reluctance of some health care systems to put health care data in the cloud. However, current trends point to the continued use of these tools and their increasingly widespread use alongside their slow adoption in health care.

- *Data science.* A term coined in 1974 with theoretical foundations that include statistics and computer science to describe a field focused on extracting new knowledge from data.[29] Typically, data scientists have trained in statistics, computer science, and linear algebra arming them with the necessary skills to wrangle Big Data and derive meaningful insights from it. In addition to the data processing described earlier in this article, data scientists explore and describe data with statistical rigor, develop and trial machine learning algorithms, and select and implement machine learning models (along with machine learning engineering counterparts) to uncover insights. Furthermore, data scientists are involved in generating descriptive analyses of Big Data sets and developing predictive and prognostic models to answer questions seeking novel findings. In health care, data scientists with additional domain knowledge can be valuable to an organization as they understand the context and nuance of data in clinical settings. As this is rarely the case, this presents an opportunity for physicians to collaborate with data scientists to enable the work.[20]
- *Machine learning.* A subfield of artificial intelligence that uses massive and multidimensional digitally archived data to generate algorithms to predict outcomes or explore data. In part 5 of this collection, Dr. Srinivas and Dr. Young artfully explain machine learning and its applications to surgical practice and research. Here we will briefly mention the types of machine learning:
  ○ *Supervised.* Labeled examples of the outcome of interest are used for model training. For example, a research team attempts to predict which patients are most likely to develop a wound infection following an appendectomy. This framing is a supervised machine learning problem assuming that the training data set has examples of patients who developed wound infection following an appendectomy. Importantly, these examples need to be labeled, meaning the wound infection is defined with a diagnosis code or other structured data element. These positive instances (of when a wound infection occurred) are used to train the model as to the pattern of data present, which the model will then use to predict future cases of wound infection.
  ○ *Unsupervised.* There are no labeled examples of the population or cohort of interest. Instead of prediction, unsupervised learning is used for clustering and

generating association rules. With clustering, unsupervised machine learning models group like instances according to their similarities and differences.
   o *Semi-supervised*. There are only a few labeled instances of the population or cohort of interest. Returning to our wound infection example, perhaps only a few positive cases of wound infection are labeled, and many cases are unlabeled (including those with and without a wound infection. In this situation, semi-supervised methods can be used to train a model on the minimal number of labeled samples available and attempt to label those instances with an unknown outcome correctly.[30]

Data visualization

Data visualization is a powerful tool for telling stories with data. Although the complexities of Big Data often hinder the user's ability to understand and analyze key concepts, data visualization techniques are well suited to showcase trends, anomalies, and insights to end users in a way that reduces cognitive load and facilitates decision-making.[31] According to data visualization pioneer Few, visualizing data should be used for sense-making and communication.[32] Indeed, data accompanied by poor visualizations risk being dismissed or misinterpreted by data consumers, including business leaders and physicians.[31,33]

In an excellent review paper, Gotz and Borland describe the unique challenges with data visualization in health care such as

- *Breadth of use.* Visualizations in health care are used for patient-level (both patient-facing and provider-facing), cohort-level, and population-level visualizations. This variety in the breadth of use requires considerations for how data are used within a visualization, the users' workflow when accessing this information, and how a visualization might change according to the context (eg, Mrs. Miller's data when viewed by her surgical oncologist and her endocrinologist).
- *Data complexity.* Data in health care are noisy, messy, and composed of various heterogenous sources, all causing challenges for data visualization. The variety of data types, such as numeric, categorical, and hierarchical elements confront those designing data visualizations. In addition, patient care is a longitudinal process where the data collected a year ago may be important to juxtapose with the data captured today. The longitudinality of data, as well as its temporal nature, are crucial to correctly visualizing health care data.
- *Statistical rigor.* Data visualization excels as rapidly finding and showing trends, commonalities, and aberrations within large data sets. However, it is not enough to show an end user in health care an "interesting" finding. Any discovery generated by data visualization must be buttressed with statistical rigor, including adequate sample size, considerations of degrees of freedom, and statistical significance.[33]

To manage these challenges, Thomas and Cook[34] provide several desiderata of data visualization tools:

- *Visual scalability*. The ability of a data visualization tool to show analyses from massive data sets quickly, reliably, and efficiently
- *Information scalability*. The ability to extract relevant findings from Big Data
- *Software scalability*. The ability of a tool to readily manage a variety of data set sizes.

Data visualization lies at the intersection of analytics and cognitive science and works closely with the field of human–computer interaction (HCI). Many excellent resources are available for those wanting additional content on capabilities and potential options of data visualization tools.

DISCUSSION
Addressing the Knowledge Gap

There is a recognized need for data management skills and training in the biomedical research community.[35] A basic understanding of these Big Data topics is necessary for surgeons to be conversant in Big Data management. As we have mentioned, a feature of Big Data is that it is challenging to manage with traditional hardware and software. Therefore, incorporating cloud computing, virtualization, and Big Data platforms is necessary. However, these Big Data tools are complex and lack the user-friendly interfaces to which nontechnical users are accustomed. Therefore, programmers or developers with experience using these open-source tools are critical to using, operating, and querying these systems.[1] This limitation challenges physicians to take full advantage of the data assets available to them—and to be appropriately involved in Big Data projects within their institution. As much research has suggested, the promise of Big Data in health care must include computers, data, and clinicians to be truly impactful. Nonclinicians cannot be left to devise and answer challenging problems in health care. Without the necessary experience and context, insights may be overlooked, or faulty conclusions may be reached.[20] By understanding Big Data management and applications, clinicians can position themselves as effective partners.[36] The aim of this article is not to make physicians into IT experts. Still, it is to provide a resource from which surgeon scientists can understand the basics of Big Data storage, management, and use to aid in conversations with the IT team, data scientists, and the health system's technology leaders.

Facilitating the Information Interchange with Information Technology

Much of the impetus for writing this article is to improve the efficiency and effectiveness of the surgical researcher: to provide surgeons with the tools to have productive conversations with the IT division to facilitate research, analysis, and the use of data-intensive applications. Depending on the size of your health system, the IT and associated divisions may include some or all the following roles:

- Executive leaders such as the chief information officer, chief medical information officer),
- Database administrators or architects,
- Business analysists,
- Data engineers, and
- Data scientists.
- Medical librarians may also act as liaisons between research teams, IT groups, and informaticians.[35]

Proactively reaching out to meet the IT team can facilitate future collaborations. The IT team is a diverse and talented group of stakeholders with wide-ranging responsibilities across a health system.

SUMMARY

A basic understanding of Big Data management is needed for surgeons to interact effectively with their IT peers. Given the advanced tools and techniques needed to manipulate and analyze Big Data, such interactions are required. As Big Data permeates health care, the continued collaboration between physicians and technical personnel will become increasingly critical. Physicians who can familiarize themselves with their technical counterparts and become facile in this domain's basic concepts and vernacular will benefit. Finally, the impact of Big Data on the day-to-day practice of medicine depends on physicians remaining "in the game" of Big Data applications.

DISCLOSURE

The author works in the health technology industry and has no conflicts related to her work and this chapter.

REFERENCES

1. Raghupathi W, Raghupathi V. Big data analytics in healthcare: promise and potential. Health Inf Sci Syst 2014;2(1). https://doi.org/10.1186/2047-2501-2-3.
2. Pramanik PK, Pal S, Mukhopadhyay M. Healthcare big data: a comprehensive overview. In research anthology on big data analytics, architectures, and applications. IGI Glob 2022;19–47. https://doi.org/10.4018/978-1-6684-3662-2.ch006.
3. RBC Capital Markets: navigating the changing face of healthcare episode. Available at: https://www.rbccm.com/en/gib/healthcare/episode/the_healthcare_data_explosion. Accessed November 18, 2022.
4. Danciu I, Cowan JD, Basford M, et al. Secondary use of clinical data: the Vanderbilt approach. J Biomed Inform 2014;52:28–35.
5. Mohammed-Rajput N, Rajput ZA, Cusack CM. Health information systems and applications. In: Finnell JT, Dixon BE, editors. Clinical Informatics study guide. Cham: Springer; 2016. p. 219–32.
6. Stobierski T. 8 steps in the data lifecycle: HBS online. Business insights blog. Available at: https://online.hbs.edu/blog/post/data-life-cycle. Accessed November 14, 2022.
7. DeWitt JG, Hampton PM. Development of a data warehouse at an academic health system: knowing a place for the first time. Acad Med 2005;80(11):1019–25.
8. Wade TD. Traits and types of health data repositories. Health Inf Sci Syst 2014;2(1):1–8.
9. Campion TR Jr, Sholle ET, Pathak J, et al. An architecture for research computing in health to support clinical and translational investigators with electronic patient data. J Am Med Inform Assoc 2022;29(4):677–85.
10. Johnson KE, Kamineni A, Fuller S, et al. How the provenance of electronic health record data matters for research: a case example using system mapping. eGEMS 2014;2(1). https://doi.org/10.13063/2327-9214.1058.
11. Curcin V. Embedding data provenance into the learning health system to facilitate reproducible research. Learn Health Syst 2017;1:2.
12. Silverstein JC, Foster IT. Computer architectures for health care and biomedicine. In: Shortliffe EH, Cimino JJ, editors. Biomedical informatics. 4th edition. London: Springer; 2014. p. 149–84. https://doi.org/10.1007/978—1-4471-4474-8_5.
13. Dhudasia MB, Grundmeier RW, Mukhopadhyay S. Essentials of data management: an overview. Pediatr Res 2021;18:1–2.
14. Famili A, Shen WM, Weber R, et al. Data preprocessing and intelligent data analysis. Intell Data Anal 1997;1(1):3–23.
15. Braunstein ML. Health care in the age of interoperability: the potential and challenges. IEEE Pulse 2018;9(5):34–6.

16. Weeks J, Pardee R. Learning to share health care data: a brief timeline of influential common data models and distributed health data networks in US health care research. eGEMs 2019;7(1):4.

17. Klann JG, Joss MA, Embree K, et al. Data model harmonization for the all of us research program: transforming i2b2 data into the OMOP common data model. PLoS One 2019;14(2):e0212463.

18. Braunstein ML. Healthcare in the age of interoperability: the promise of fast healthcare interoperability resources. IEEE Pulse 2018;9(6):24–7.

19. Azeroual O. Data wrangling in database systems: purging of dirty data. Data 2020;5(2):50.

20. Celi LA, Davidzon G, Johnson AE, et al. Bridging the health data divide. J Med Internet Res 2016;18(12):e325.

21. Evans RS, Lloyd JF, Pierce LA. Clinical use of an enterprise data warehouse. AMIA Annu Symp Proc 2012;2012:189–98.

22. Nargesian F, Zhu E, Miller RJ, et al. Data lake management: challenges and opportunities. Proc VLDB Endowment 2019;12(12):1986–9.

23. Kidd C. Data storage explained: data lake vs warehouse vs database. BMC Blogs. Available at: https://www.bmc.com/blogs/data-lake-vs-data-warehouse-vs-database-whats-the-difference/. Accessed November 15, 2022.

24. Kohn MA, Newman TB, Hulley SB. Data management. In: Hulley SB, Cummings ST, Warren SB, et al, editors. Designing clinical research. 3rd edition. Philadelphia: Lippincott Williams & Wilkins; 2007. p. 257–69.

25. Sumathi S, Esakkirajan S. Overview of database management system. In: Fundamentals of relational database management systems. Springer; 2007. p. 1–30.

26. Leavitt N. Will NoSQL databases live up to their promise? Computer 2010; 43(2):12–4.

27. Pavlenko E, Strech D, Langhof H. Implementation of data access and use procedures in clinical data warehouses. a systematic review of literature and publicly available policies. BMC Med Inform Decis Mak 2020;20(1):1–3.

28. What is data lineage? IBM. Available at: https://www.ibm.com/topics/data-lineage. Accessed November 19, 2022.

29. Borjigin C, Zhang C. Data science: trends, perspectives, and prospects. Res Square 2021. https://doi.org/10.21203/rs.3.rs-1014621/v2.

30. Iavindrasana J, Cohen G, Depeursinge A, et al. Clinical data mining: a review. Yearb Med Inform 2009;18(01):121–33.

31. Khasnabish S, Burns Z, Couch M, et al. Best practices for data visualization: creating and evaluating a report for an evidence-based fall prevention program. J Am Med Inform Assoc 2020;27(2):308–14.

32. Few S. Data visualization for human perception. In: The encyclopedia of human-computer interaction. 2nd edition. Interaction Design Foundation; 2014.

33. Gotz D, Borland D. Data-driven healthcare: challenges and opportunities for interactive visualization. IEEE Comput Graph Appl 2016;36(3):90–6.

34. Thomas JJ, Cook KA. A visual analytics agenda. IEEE Comput Graph Appl 2006; 26(1):10–3.

35. Read KB. Adapting data management education to support clinical research projects in an academic medical center. J Med Libr Assoc 2019;107(1):89–97.

36. Charow R, Jeyakumar T, Younus S, et al. Artificial intelligence education programs for health care professionals: scoping review. JMIR Med Educ 2021; 7(4):e31043.

Privacy, Data Sharing, and Other Legal Considerations

Jodi Cramer, BA, JD, LLM*

KEYWORDS

- Data • Privacy • Data sharing • HIPAA • FERPA • FTC Act

KEY POINTS

- The United States has a patchwork of privacy laws.
- Data privacy is required to be protected differently depending on the state and the sector.
- The same data can be protected under different statutes depending on the entity storing the data.

KEY/ESSENTIAL HEADINGS

- The privacy/data sharing framework in the United States is a patchwork of sector-based Federal laws and a myriad of state laws.
- The Framework is complicated and difficult to navigate.
- Not all health information is protected the same.

DISCUSSION

The concept of privacy in regards to health information dates back to ancient Greece. The earliest version of the Hippocratic Oath states, "Whatever I see or hear in the lives of my patients, whether in connection with my professional practice or not, which ought not to be spoken of outside, I will keep secret, as considering all such things to be private."[1] In the modern version of the Hippocratic Oath, the language has been updated to state, "I will respect the privacy of my patients, for their problems are not disclosed to me that the world may know."[2]

The same concept as expressed in both versions of the Hippocratic Oath has carried over to the legal system. There is a specific civil litigation privilege that allows for the protection of doctor-patient information during the litigation process. Although this privilege is not engrained in common law, it has been codified in some form in all states.[3]

Attorney, United States Coast Guard, Washington, DC, USA
* Corresponding author. 2703 Martin Luther King Junior Avenue, SE STOP 7000, Washington, DC 20593.
E-mail address: Jodi.cramer@gmail.com

Surg Clin N Am 103 (2023) 347–356
https://doi.org/10.1016/j.suc.2022.12.003
0039-6109/23/Published by Elsevier Inc.
surgical.theclinics.com

Privacy in the United States is complicated. It is a framework of both state and Federal laws, and case law precedents. The statutes apply to specific sectors such as health care, financial, education, and child protection. This patchwork of statutes and case law has created an unstable environment to ensure that privacy rights are protected. Other countries have taken a more comprehensive approach to their privacy framework, providing more stability and stricter guidelines. Although in the United States, privacy depends on the state one lives, and the latest ruling of the Supreme Court.

Before June 2022, there was a constitutional right to privacy. This was found in the 4th, 5th, 9th, and 14th Amendments to the Constitution. In Griswald v. Connecticut,[4] the Supreme Court determined that the penumbra of additional rights, not specifically articulated in the Constitution under the 9th Amendment, combined with the more specific rights to privacy spelled out in the 1st, 4th, and 5th Amendments created a "zone of privacy." In 1973, in the landmark case of Roe v. Wade,[5] the Supreme Court determined that there was a right to privacy in the 14th Amendment. In June 2022, the Supreme Court overturned Roe v Wade in Dobbs v. Jackson Women's Health Organization,[6] uprooting a Constitutional right to privacy.

Unlike the legal framework for privacy over one's body, Federal laws for data privacy stem not from case law but from statute. Congress has chosen to regulate the financial, health care, and education sectors in regards to data privacy. Through the deceptive trade practice section of the Federal Trade Commission (FTC) Act, the FTC has been able to provide limited regulation over consumer data.[7] This provision of the FTC Act does not provide specific rules on the collection and use of consumer data. Many other countries have developed a legal process that regulates the use of all privacy data such as the General Data Protection Regulation (GDPR) in the European Union.[8]

Several states such as California,[9] Virginia,[10] and Colorado[11] have enacted data privacy laws that mirror the GDPR. Unlike the GDPR, which covers all types of data privacy regardless of sector, the state laws only apply to consumer data. However, California is currently publishing additional regulations that would extend its data privacy requirements to human resource data and other types of data not covered by Federal regulations.[12] Other states have less comprehensive laws, but add additional requirements such as breach notification. There have been many attempts by Congress to create a comprehensive data privacy framework. Currently, there is a bipartisan bill, that has passed the House. It is unclear if it will receive the 60 votes needed in the Senate.[13] The precipice for the current bill is to regulate technology companies that currently collect and use personal data in ways that are buried in multi-page terms of service agreement that is rarely read and routinely updated. Although individual users have technically consented to the collection and use of their data many have little knowledge of what is being collected and how it is being used.

Not only are companies collecting and using personal data they are also selling it to third-party data brokers who buy and sell data on the open market. Data brokers not only buy and sell data but they aggregate data from multiple sources allowing them to sell more detailed profiles of individuals.[14] This ability to aggregate data allows buyers to receive data profiles that were put together without the individual's consent. Artificial intelligence is then applied to the data profile to develop strategies to convince individuals to buy products or to support a specific political position or candidate. This methodology was used by the Russian government to influence the 2016 presidential election.[14]

With the addition of smart devices, the data being collected on individuals is expeditiously increasing. Data brokers can track location, heart rates, and reproductive cycles. Big data is no longer limited to e-mail messages, Internet activity, and social media posts.[14]

The current legal framework does little to protect against the growing collection and exploitation of personal data. The US sector-based approach does provide protection for some health information, whereas other health information can be bought and sold to the highest bidder. There is no legal prohibition from buying and selling health information obtained from a smart device such as a personal cardiac reader or a smartwatch. Yet, that health information could be just as sensitive as data contained in medical records.

Health information is protected mainly by three different federal statutes: The Health Insurance Portability and Accountability Act (HIPAA),[15] The Family Education Rights and Privacy Act (FERPA),[16] and the FTC Act.[7] In addition, health data is regulated by the Common Rule when used in human subject research.[17] The Americans with Disabilities Act prohibits the disclosure of health information by employers.[18] If the health data are part of a federal government information system, it is protected by additional statutes. Each statute has different rules for the protection and disclosure of information.

Health Insurance Portability and Accountability Act

HIPAA was enacted in 1996 to provide for the protection and transferability of certain health care information.[15] It was later amended through the Health Information Technology for Economic and Clinical Health Act of 2009 (HITECH), which granted authority to the Department of Health and Human Services (HHS) to promulgate regulations for privacy and security as well as the regulatory authority to enforce those provisions. The regulations are divided into three different parts: The HIPAA Privacy Rule, The HIPAA Security Rule, and The HIPAA Enforcement Rule. The Privacy Rule outlines how health care data can be released and to whom. The Security Rule outlines specific administrative, technical, and physical controls to protect health care data. The Enforcement Rule grants authority to HHS to assess fines when the Privacy and Security Rules are violated. In addition, HIPAA prohibits the sale of protected health information (PHI).[19–22]

Many believe that HIPAA applies to all health or medical data, but that is not the case. HIPAA only applies to health information at a covered entity or business associate. The HIPAA regulations at 45 C.F.R. §160.103 defines health information as, "any information, including genetic information, whether oral or recorded in any form or medium, that: (1) Is created or received by a health care provider, health plan, public health authority, employer, life insurer, school or university, or health care clearinghouse; and (2) Relates to the past, present, or future physical or mental health or condition of an individual; the provision of health care to an individual; or the past, present, or future payment for the provision of health care to an individual." HIPAA further defines PHI as "individually identifiable health information: (1) Except as provided in paragraph (2) of this definition, that is: (i) Transmitted by electronic media; (ii) Maintained in electronic media; or (iii) Transmitted or maintained in any other form or medium. (2) PHI excludes individually identifiable health information: (i) In education records covered by the Family Educational Rights and Privacy Act, as amended, 20 U.S.C. 1232g; (ii) In records described at 20 U.S.C. 1232g(a) (4) (B) (iv); (iii) In employment records held by a covered entity in its role as employer; and (iv) Regarding a person who has been deceased for more than 50 years."[22] The definition of health information does not include medical data collected by the Internet of things devices and stored on smartphones or in the cloud such as devices that monitor heartbeats, cardiac monitors, and drug monitors, except from when that information is incorporated into the records of those entities in part 1 of the definition.

In addition to meeting the definition of health information, the data must be created or received by a "covered entity" or a "business associate." A covered entity is defined in 45 C.F.R. §160.103 as "(1) A health plan. (2) A health care clearinghouse. (3) A health care provider who transmits any health information in electronic form in connection with a transaction covered by this subchapter." A "business associate" is defined in the same provision as "(i) A Health Information Organization, E-prescribing Gateway, or other person that provides data transmission services with respect to PHI to a covered entity and that requires access on a routine basis to such PHI. (ii) A person that offers a personal health record to one or more individuals on behalf of a covered entity. (iii) A subcontractor that creates, receives, maintains, or transmits PHI on behalf of the business associate."[22]

Any entity not falling under the definitions of a 'covered entity" or "business associate" is not required to follow the HIPAA Privacy and Security Rules. This includes any HIPAA information once it is properly released to another entity. For example, one of the allowable releases under the HIPAA Privacy Rule is to military commanders for readiness determinations of military personnel. Once the information is transmitted to the commander. it is no longer protected under HIPAA.[20]

The HIPAA Privacy Rule outlines how and to whom health information can be shared and the consent and notice provisions for individuals. Specifically, it limits who can access health information while allowing health data to flow between those who are authorized to have access. Other than to the individual (except for some psychiatric notes and court proceedings) there are few required releases (public health); most are permissible. It also requires that the individual receive notice of what information is collected and to whom the information is released. Even when permissible an individual or entity should only release the minimal amount necessary for the specific purpose. For example, a health care provider only needs to disclose to a health care insurer the minimal amount of information needed to process the insurance. An individual can also consent to share their records with any individual or entity.[20]

The HIPAA Privacy Rule does allow for the release of HIPAA-protected information if the information has been de-identified, as once the data has been de-identified, it is not considered HIPAA PHI. Per the Rule, there are two ways to de-identify data. (1) To use an expert to de-identify the data. Experts do not have to be experts in health care. (2) Is to remove 18 specific fields. Removing the specific fields is called the "safe harbor" method. It is important to note, that if the data is re-identified it becomes protected again. De-identified data can be publicly released and is a way to share information without infringing on an individual's privacy.[20]

The HIPAA Privacy Rule is the only regulation/statute that specifically outlines how to de-identify information. Other regulations such as the GDPR discuss de-identifying data or in the case of the GDPR–pseudonymization, Other statutes also consider de-identified information to be no longer protected.[8]

The HIPAA Security Rule outlines specific technical, administrative, and physical controls needed to protect health care data. Although most of the controls are similar to those in commercial security standards such as NIST 800-53[23] (which outlines technical, physical, and administrative controls for both government and commercial entities), it was an early adopter of requiring encryption at rest and transit.[21]

HIPAA also has specific requirements to report data breaches. All breaches from a covered entity of over 500 individuals must be reported to HHS within 60 days. If the breach involved the data of over 500 individuals in a particular state it must be reported to the media within 60 days. A covered entity must notify the individual of any breach (no matter the number of impacted individuals) within 60 days, that time is extended to 90 days if there are more than 10 invalid addresses. Within 60 days of the end of the year, covered entities need to report a yearly tally of all breaches to HHS. Business associates are only required to report a breach to the covered entity within 60 days.[24]

In addition to HIPAA, there are a plethora of state laws that cover the same or similar information. In the US system, Federal law usually pre-empts state law, unless the state law is stricter than the Federal law. When that happens, the Federal law applies in that jurisdiction. Many states had laws before HIPAA was enacted. HIPAA uses the term "contrary" to define a state law that is not aligned with HIPAA. "Contrary" is defined as" when used to compare a provision of State law to a standard, requirement, or implementation specification adopted under this subchapter, means: (1) A covered entity or business associate would find it impossible to comply with both the State and Federal requirements; or (2) The provision of State law stands as an obstacle to the accomplishment and execution of the full purposes and objectives of part C of title XI of the Act, section 264 of Public Law 104-191, or sections 13400-13424 of Public Law 111-5, as applicable." State law applies when it is "more stringent" which is defined as: "in the context of a comparison of a provision of State law and a standard, requirement, or implementation specification adopted under subpart E of part 164 of this subchapter, a State law that meets one or more of the following criteria". Criteria include greater notification and greater access to information for the individual.[22] As the states have some enforcement ability under HIPAA, states had to review their laws to determine which provisions still apply or which were superseded by HIPAA. As such, it is important for anyone who collects health information to consult their state law as well as the Federal law. In some cases, states may include information not protected under HIPAA, such as health information retained by employers or mobile devices as PHI.

Before HIPAA, there were two Federal laws that protected the release of information on drug and alcohol abuse. The Comprehensive Alcohol Abuse and Alcoholism Prevention, Treatment, and Rehabilitation Act Amendments of 1979,[25] Drug Abuse Prevention, Treatment, and Rehabilitation Act of 1979[26] and the implementing regulations entitled The Substance Abuse Confidentiality Regulations[27] to require that organizations that receive federal funding only release personal information about substance abuse patients with consent. There are a few exceptions such as medical emergencies, research, audits, child abuse reporting, and a court order.

Federal Trade Commission Act

Section 5 of the FTC Act allows the FTC to enforce unfair or deceptive practices in the marketplace, The FTC uses this provision to regulate consumer data privacy in the United States; this includes health data. In fact, even data protected under HIPAA is subjected to the unfair/deceptive trade practices of the FTC Act.[28] As it was written to protect against unfair/deceptive trade practices it is not a comprehensive privacy statute. There are two prongs to the deceptive practices: (1) under the "deceptive" prong the company has misrepresented its practices, which requires that such a representation has, in fact, been made; (2) and under the "unfairness" prong, the company's poor data practice is "unfair" to the consumer, because it: (a) causes substantial harm, (b) that does not outweigh benefits, and (c) the harm is one that consumers cannot reasonably avoid.[7]

An example of a deceptive trade practice is if a privacy notice for a fitness tracker states it will not sell a user's data yet the company sells it to a data broker. This was the issue in the enforcement against Facebook, where Facebook was found to have engaged in deceptive trade practices by releasing data to third parties in violation of the notice given to users. Facebook was fined $5 billion for the violation, one of the largest fines ever issued by the Federal government.[29] The FTC Act does not require consent or notification to share data. It only requires that an entity does not deceive the consumer. So, if a company states that they will sell the data, or share it with unlimited third parties, it is in compliance with the statute.

The FTC also promulgated a rule that requires the reporting of the breach of non-HIPAA health records. The notification and timelines are very similar to those for HIPAA records, yet the reporting is to the FTC as opposed to HHS. The FTC rule applies to "personal health record vendors" who are "an entity, other than a HIPAA-covered entity or an entity to the extent that it engages in activities as a business associate of a HIPAA-covered entity, that offers or maintains a personal health record." The rule defines a "personal health record" as "an electronic record of PHR identifiable health information on an individual that can be drawn from multiple sources and that is managed, shared, and controlled by or primarily for the individual."[30] The FTC in a policy statement has determined that the rule applies to health apps such as fitness trackers and blood sugar monitors if it pulls information for multiple sources, even if the other sources do not contain health information.[31]

There are also several states that have more stringent laws that govern consumer data. The most significant of the state laws is the California Consumer Privacy Act (CCPA). The CCPA was modeled after the EU's GDPR, but unlike the GDPR it only applies to consumer data (although it is being expanded to employment data) of residents of the State of California (even if the data is stored outside of California), for companies that have gross revenue over $25 million, collects information on over 50,000 individuals, or derives 50% of their profits from selling consumer information. It does not apply to organizations regulated by HIPAA. The law requires notice of data sharing and the ability to opt out. It also allows individuals to obtain information about their data and with whom it was shared.[9] If the current national privacy bill passes the Senate and is signed into law, it will supersede state laws such as the CCPA.[13]

Family Education Rights and Privacy Act

As outlined in the definition of PHI under the HIPAA regulations, health information protected by FERPA is not protected by HIPAA. This is the case with student treatment records at post-secondary medical clinics. Student medical records at a university hospital would be subject to HIPAA as it is a covered entity and its focus is to treat the public. Records known as "treatment records" that are kept in medical clinics are only releasable to a parent without the student's consent if the student is a dependent, it is a health emergency where informing the parents will prevent or assist with the emergency, or if it is a drug or alcohol issue for students under the age of 21.[32]

Treatment records can also be released to other medical professionals who are treating the student or a health care provider of the student's choice. When the records are transferred to a covered entity, the transferred records are covered under HIPAA, whereas the copy at the medical clinic remains protected under FERPA.[32] Any other release of student treatment records converts the records into "education records" which can be released without consent for numerous reasons including law enforcement, for financial aid, and other administrative purposes.[33]

Human Subject Research

When identified personal information is used in research it is considered human subject research, making it subject to the "Common Rule" for federally funded research projects, and similar schemas for other projects. The common rule was recently updated to clarify how consent works with personal data in research. The general rule is that to conduct research on human subjects there needs to be informed consent. Informed consent, as outlined in 45 C.F.R. 46.116 adds the reasonable person standard, which requires notice to be not only written in a way that can be understood by a study subject, but must include information that a reasonable person would need to consent to participate in the study.[17] The regulation in the same section also allows for broad consent for the storage, maintenance and secondary use of data or biospecimens. Broad consent still has a notice requirement, however, it is limited to: a general description of the research, a description of the data or biospecimens and what institutions might conduct additional research, the period of time the data or biospecimens will be kept, notice that subjects will or won't be informed of additional research, and notice that subjects will or will not be informed of the study results.[17]

An Institutional Review Board (IRB) may waive the consent requirement under section 116 of the regulation for one of the following conditions: (1) The only identifiable information would be the consent form. (2) The study is of less than minimum risk to the subject and there are no procedures involved in the research that would otherwise require consent. 3. The study participants are part of a cultural group whose culture is not accustom to signing forms. It is unclear how this provision will apply in states where consent is required to collect or share data. It some cases the data required for the research, may have passed through so many entities it will be impossible to determine the original collection point and if consent was given.[17]

In addition, there is specific information that is exempt from the definition of research (and therefore the need for consent) per 44 C.F.R. 46.104. The most significant of the examples is for secondary research. Secondary research is not considered research when the data or biospecimens are: 1. Available to the public. 2. De-identified. 3. Regulated under HIPAA. 4. Uses government or government-collected information that was collected for a non-research purpose.[17] There will need to be further guidance to determine if available to the public includes data sold by data brokers.

HIPAA allows for protected health data to be released for research purposes if an IRB or privacy board has approved or granted a waiver of informed consent. In addition, the covered entity must review the research to determine that the information is required to establish a research protocol, ensure PHI not be removed from the covered entity, and the information is necessary to conduct the research. In addition, if the research is on deceased individuals it must be documented at the time of the request.[20]

If the research or secondary research is being performed at a covered entity and the information meets the definition of PHI it will be required to follow HIPAA.[22] If the research is conducted at a non-covered entity and it combines multiple sources of information, one being health information then the FTC's health information breach rule is applicable.[30]

US Federal Framework

Information retained by the US Government has additional statutory protection in the form of the Privacy Act of 1974 and the E-Government Act of 2002. Personal information that is contained in a system of records, which is a filing system where the information is retrieved by a personal identifier (such as name, number, or symbol) is protected by the Privacy Act. Under the Privacy Act, the Federal government must publish a notice, called a System of Records Notice (SORN) in the Federal Register which contains what information is being collected, under what authority, where it is being stored, and under what conditions it can be released. Information can always be released to the individual or to a third party with consent unless there is an exemption published in the SORN (these include law enforcement and other sensitive systems). In addition, there are 12 statutory exceptions that allow for release of the information without consent. These include: to agency employees, for Freedom of Information Act purposes, law enforcement, statistical research, emergency response, and via a court order.[34] The Privacy Act and HIPAA have similar notice and consent requirements, so most Privacy Act systems are also HIPAA compliant or can be with a few adjustments.

In addition, the E-Government Act[35] that includes the Federal Information Security Management Act requires that agency implement specific administrative, technical, and physical controls as outlined by the National Institute on Standards and Technology (NIST).[36] The current controls are outlined in NIST 800-53, although agencies can enact stricter controls. In addition, the E-Government Act requires agencies to post a privacy impact assessment on all IT systems that contain personally identifiable information (PII) and requires the Office of Budget and Management to promulgate regulations to define PII and processes to report breaches.[35]

General Data Privacy Regulation

The GDPR is the EU's comprehensive privacy regulation that covers all collections of personal information with a few exceptions for law enforcement and household activities. It has specific guidelines for the collection and use of data. One of the requirements is that data may only leave the EU if there are binding corporate rules, standard contract clause, consent of the individual, or an adequacy determination by the EU of the other country's privacy framework.[8] The United States has not met the requirements for a nationwide adequacy determination. As such, the EU and the United States have developed a framework that allows US companies to certify to meeting specific privacy controls in exchange for the ability to transfer data from the EU. The first two frameworks were ruled to be insufficient by an EU court.[37] However, in March 2022, the United States and the EU announced a new framework.[38]

SUMMARY

The legal framework to protect data in the United States is a sector-based patchwork of Federal and state laws. The rules for protecting and sharing data depend on the type of data, the entity collecting the data, and any additional state laws. HIPAA, The FTC Act, and FERPA are all very different. When health data are used in human subject research there are additional requirements for using the data. It is important to also review any applicable state laws that may impact the collection or sharing of data. If Congress passes a new privacy statute it will synchronize some of the current state laws and provide additional regulations for consumer data. However, it does not look like the United States will adopt an all-encompassed GDPR-like statute and instead will stick with its sector-based approach to data privacy.

DISCLOSURE

The authors have nothing to disclose. But add: "J. Cramer is a government civilian for the US Coast Guard. The views presented in this article are her own and do not necessarily represent the views of the Department of Homeland Security or the US Coast Guard."

REFERENCES

1. Hippocratis. Hippocratic Oath. Secondary Hippocratic Oath, Available at: https://www.nlm.nih.gov/hmd/greek/greek_oath.html. Accessed July 16, 2022.

2. Lasagn L. The Hippocratic Oath: Modern Version. Secondary The Hippocratic Oath: Modern Version 1964, Available at: https://www.pbs.org/wgbh/nova/doctors/oath_modern.html. Accessed July 16, 2022.
3. Team WD. Doctor-patient privilege. Secondary Doctor-patient privilege 2020, Available at: https://www.law.cornell.edu/wex/doctor-patient_privilege. Accessed July 16, 2022.
4. Griswald v. Conneticut, 381 U.S. 479. U.S.: Supreme Court, 1965.
5. Roe v. Wade, 410 U.S. 113: Supreme Court, 1973.
6. Dobbs v. Jackson Women's health organization, 587 U.S. _____ (No. 19-1392): Supreme Court, 2022.
7. Federal Trade Commission Act, 1914.
8. General Data Protection Regulation. In: Union E, ed., 2016.
9. California Consumer Privacy Act. In: California, ed., 2018.
10. Virginia Consumer Data Protection Act, 2021.
11. Colorado Privacy Act, 2021.
12. California Privacy Rights Act, 2020.
13. Lima C. House panel advances major privacy bill. Washington Post: Striking a Long-Awaited Grand Bargain; 2022.
14. Sherman J. Data brokers are a threat to democracy, 2021, Wired. Available at: www.wired.com/story/opinion-data-brokers-are-a-threat-to-democracy/. Accessed July 16, 2022.
15. Health Insurance Portability and Accountability Act of 1996 § Public. Law 1996; 104-191.
16. Family Educational Rights and Privacy Act § 20 U.S.C. § 1232g (1974).
17. Human Subject Research § 45 C.F.R. 46 (Department of Health and Human Services ed.).
18. The Americans with Disabilities Act of 1990 § Public. Law 1990;101-336.
19. Health Information Technology for. Economic and Clinical Health Act of 2009 § Public. Law 2009;111-5.
20. HIPAA Privacy Rule § 45 C.F.R. 160, 164 (Department of Health and Human Services ed.).
21. HIPAA Security Rule § 45 C.F.R. 160,164 (Department of Health and Human Services ed.).
22. HIPAA General Regulation § 45 C.F.R. 160.
23. National Institute of Science and Technology. NIST Special Publication 800-53, Security and Privacy Controls for Information Systems and Organizations rev 5.
24. HIPAA Brach Notification Rule § 45 CFR §§ 164.400-414 (Department of Health and Human Services ed.).
25. Comprehensive Alcohol Abuse, Alcoholism Prevention. Treatment, and Rehabilitation Act Amendments of 1979 §. Public Law 1979;96-180.
26. Drug Abuse Prevention, Treatment, and Rehabilitation Act of 1979 § Public Law 96-104 (1979).
27. Substance Abuse Confidentiality Regulations § 42 CFR Part 2.
28. Services FTCaTDoHaH. Sharing Consumer Health Information? Secondary Sharing Consumer Health Information?. Available at: https://www.hhs.gov/sites/default/files/pdf-0219_sharing-health-info-hippa-ftcact%20508.pdf.
29. Commission, F. T. (2019, July 24, 2019). *FTC Imposes $5 Billion Penalty and Sweeping New Privacy Restrictions on Facebook.* Available at: https://www.ftc.gov/news-events/news/press-releases/2019/07/ftc-imposes-5-billion-penalty-sweeping-new-privacy-restrictions-facebook. Accessed July 16, 2022.

30. Health Breach Notification Rule § 16 CFR Part 318 (Federal Trade Commission ed., 2022).
31. *STATEMENT OF THE COMMISSION On Breaches by Health Apps and Other Connected Devices.* (2021). Retrieved from https://www.ftc.gov/system/files/documents/public_statements/1596364/statement_of_the_commission_on_breaches_by_health_apps_and_other_connected_devices.pdf. Accessed July 16, 2022.
32. *Joint Guidance on the Application of the Family Educational Rights and Privacy Act (FERPA) And the Health Insurance Portability and Accountability Act of 1996 (HIPAA) To Student Health Records*(2019). Retrieved from https://www.hhs.gov/sites/default/files/2019-hipaa-ferpa-joint-guidance.pdf. Accessed July 16, 2022.
33. Family Educational Rights and Privacy Act Regulations § 34 C.F.R. Part 99.
34. Privacy Act of 1974 § Public Law 93-579 (1974).
35. E-Government Act of 2002 § Public. Law 2002;107-347.
36. Federal Information Security. Management Act 2002.
37. Privacy Shield Program Overview. Secondary Privacy Shield Program Overview. Available at: https://www.privacyshield.gov/Program-Overview.
38. House, T.W. (2022). *FACT SHEET: United States and European Commission Announce Trans-Atlantic Data Privacy Framework* https://www.whitehouse.gov/briefing-room/statements-releases/2022/03/25/fact-sheet-united-states-and-european-commission-announce-trans-atlantic-data-privacy-framework/. Accessed July 16, 2022.

Impact of Digital Health upon the Surgical Patient Experience: The Patient as Consumer

Heather L. Evans, MD, MS*, Joseph Scalea, MD

KEYWORDS

- Digital health • Surgery • MHealth • Remote patient monitoring

KEY POINTS

- Digital Health is a broad term referring to general applications for health and fitness to the use of monitoring apps, with or without wireless-connected devices, for diagnosis and monitoring in the setting of clinical care.
- The growth of telehealth services has substantially increased the acceptability of applying digital health interventions such as remote patient monitoring to guide decision-making, but the use in surgical patients is still early.
- Patients undergoing surgery may benefit from the incorporation of mHealth applications and online platforms for perioperative education, prehabilitation, and postoperative care coordination. However, optimal implementation and sustained use of apps and devices is dependent upon effective stakeholder engagement and user feedback integration.
- Features of digital health that may improve the surgical patient experience in the future include social networking and gamification to achieve perioperative goals, personalized alerts and treatment recommendations for optimal outcomes, and the ongoing shift toward ubiquitous monitoring.

INTRODUCTION

Digital health holds promise to expand the range of services available to prepare patients before surgery and to support their postoperative recovery. Patients undergoing surgical procedures, no matter how minor, face uncertainty and risk. The need to rapidly understand clinical circumstances and surgical options, entrust their well-being to a new provider, and adapt to previously unknown, but well-established

Dr. Evans is a member of the scientific advisory board of Crely, Inc.
Dr. Scalea owns stock and is the founder of MediGO, Inc., a digital health company, and MissionGO, Inc., an unmanned aircraft company.
Department of Surgery, Medical University of South Carolina, 96 Jonathan Lucas Street, CSB 417, Charleston, SC 29425, USA
* Corresponding author.
E-mail address: evanshe@musc.edu

Surg Clin N Am 103 (2023) 357–368
https://doi.org/10.1016/j.suc.2022.11.006
0039-6109/23/© 2022 Elsevier Inc. All rights reserved.
surgical.theclinics.com

procedures, places surgical patients in unfamiliar territory. As our society has become more reliant on electronic media for dissemination of education, news, and commerce, patients now routinely seek medical information online and may present to the surgical clinic as savvy digital customers. It is now incumbent upon surgeons to understand the digital health marketplace and to integrate available digital health tools into their practice to meet the growing needs of surgical patients.

This article outlines the scope of digital health and its clinical relevance to surgical care, with a special emphasis on patient-facing technologies. Areas to be explored include health and wellness self-tracking apps, provider-prescribed remote patient monitoring, and new avenues for health care communication and education. Controversies in the patient-centered use of digital health in surgical care, as well as barriers to adoption and sustainability are examined.

Finally, we propose future possibilities for the application of digital health to improve the patient experience and surgical outcomes.

Scope of Digital Health

The Federal Drug Administration (FDA) has been tasked with providing regulatory policy and oversight for "digital health." The broad scope of digital health includes categories such as mobile health (mHealth), health information technology (HIT), wearable devices, telehealth and telemedicine, and personalized medicine. To the patient as consumer, the experience of digital health spans from general applications for health and fitness to the use of monitoring apps, with or without wireless-connected devices, for diagnosis and monitoring in the setting of clinical care. Over time, digital communications are augmenting, and in some cases replacing, traditional in-person and telephonic encounters; patients may opt-in to access their medical records via patient portals and their providers via telehealth messaging and/or video visits. Outside of the direct awareness of the patient as consumer, all of this technology relies upon use of secure networks, cloud-based storage, and various levels of interoperability between systems, as well as the use of big data for the development and application of algorithmic decision support.

Digital health also critically extends to the direct-to-patient marketing services. Even outside of the context of medical care delivery, patients are increasingly bombarded with opportunities to self-educate and self-track their health, with the promise of self-improvement. According to industry estimates in 2017, 325,000 health care applications were available on smartphones, which equates to an expected 3.7 billion mobile health application downloads that year by smartphone users worldwide.[1] In 2019, 60% of mobile phone owners worldwide used their smartphones for health education and information seeking.[2] The line between "software as a medical device" and advisory or educational apps is somewhat unclear, but generally the use of a smartphone or artificial intelligence algorithms for medical decision-making and diagnosis requires a higher level of regulatory approval. As such, many of the apps directly marketed to consumers are categorized as "wellness" or "health education" programs, which do not purport to provide personalized diagnosis or medical care. However, many of these apps use gamification, the application of typical elements of game playing (eg, point scoring, competition with others, rules of play) as a marketing technique to elicit initial engagement with a product or service, and to encourage users to achieve a desired outcome. It is important to acknowledge that most medical education apps and other digital resources available on the Internet are outside the scope of regulation by the FDA, and patients should be advised to be savvy consumers, using only resources curated by trusted sources.

CLINICAL RELEVANCE OF DIGITAL HEALTH IN SURGICAL CARE

The increasing availability of digital health resources has substantially impacted the delivery of care in surgical specialties. The exponential growth of telehealth, including remote patient monitoring, as well as increased access to surgical information on the Internet brings a new paradigm to the surgeon-patient relationship. In this section, the influence of digital health tools on a shift from provider-centered to patient-centered surgical care will be considered.

Conversely, the potential impact of provider-prescribed digital health interventions will be reviewed.

Growth of Telehealth in Surgery

The explosion of telehealth, whether video visits or store-and-forward messaging, has provided patients with unprecedented access to surgical providers. Although not all surgeons have continued to use video visits as a means to provide initial consultations or postoperative follow-up, during the COVID-19 pandemic, televisits provided critical access for patients to maintain continuity of care. Owing to the loosening of regulatory limitations on inter-state care delivery and facilitation of remote care reimbursement during the public health emergency, the implementation of telehealth was fast-tracked as a primary means of initiating and continuing surgical care in a time of resource scarcity. Video visits became much more accepted by both patients and surgeons during this time, but even before the pandemic, the use of asynchronous communications via electronic medical record patient portals grew substantially. Nearly 40 percent of individuals nationwide accessed a patient portal in 2020, a 13 percentage point increase since 2014.[3] About six in 10 patient portal users exchanged secure messages with their health care provider in 2020, representing a 10 percentage point increase from 2017. Current patient drivers for maintenance and expansion of telehealth services include ongoing demand for access to care, convenience of scheduling, and avoidance of transportation-related costs. Durable provider and system incentives focus on efficiency and expansion of care delivery, resulting in consumer satisfaction. Surgeons have a unique opportunity to employ telehealth for straightforward postoperative visits, as most occur within the global period and reimbursement for the encounter is irrelevant. Harkey and colleagues showed similar patient satisfaction, but increased convenience among patients randomized to telehealth follow-up visits versus traditional in-person visits after low-risk surgery.[4] Furthermore, this was achieved with more direct contact with patients and greater care efficiency.[5] However, these benefits are balanced by barriers to telehealth adoption and sustainability, including patient lack of broadband and device access, technology education, and reversion to old interstate medical care compacts that prevent provision of health care across state lines. Lack of payment parity and limit to the physical examination required in some surgical disease processes may limit the application of telehealth visits for initial consultation. Alternatively, patients who live in rural and/or remote areas with limited access to advanced tertiary care for complex surgical conditions may benefit from consultation using imaging and laboratory screening.[6] Surgical oncology consultations may benefit from a hybrid use of telemedicine to allow distant family or caregivers to participate synchronously in treatment discussions.[7] The integration of telehealth into a surgical encounter is a work-in-progress.

Remote Patient Monitoring

Another growing area of telehealth in surgical care is the use of physiologic and other patient generated health data for pre- and postoperative symptom surveillance.

Remote patient monitoring (RPM) refers specifically to the use of digital technology to capture and analyze patients' physiological data, such as blood pressure, glucose levels, and lung function. By contrast, remote therapeutic monitoring focuses on non-physiological data, such as patient adherence and reported pain levels. For the purposes of this review, the term "remote patient monitoring" will be used synonymously for both kinds of monitoring, referring to the extension of patient data acquisition and transmission outside of in-person care. In the context of surgical care delivery, RPM may be applied along the duration of the surgical care encounter, from working toward prehabilitation goals, to use in the hospital to assess for postoperative milestone achievement, and to the post-discharge care coordination phase in triage of

postoperative symptoms and personalized follow-up scheduling. The patient may leverage smartphone hardware and wireless-connected sensors to record and transmit data from their devices via an institutionally-sponsored portal or third-party platform for centralized review. Examples of RPM relevant to surgical care include surgical wound monitoring with digital photographs and symptom reports for patients at high risk of surgical site infection;[8] preoperative weight measurement, dietary logs, and activity monitoring for prehabilitation;[9] postoperative heart rate and rhythm monitoring, weight measurement, and pulse oximetry after cardiac surgery;[10] immunosuppression medication adherence after solid organ transplantation.[11]

There is a growing body of literature on the impact of RPM on surgical outcomes facilitated by mHealth apps and wearable devices. A systematic review of mHealth use to track surgical patients after hospital discharge revealed that exposure to mHealth was associated with fewer emergency department visits (odds ratio 0.42, [C.I. 0.23–0.79]) and readmissions (odds ratio 0.47 [C.I. 0.29–0.77]) as well as accelerated improvements in quality of life after surgery.[12] A randomized controlled trial of activity monitoring and bidirectional text messaging on the rate of discharge to home and clinical outcomes in patients receiving hip or knee arthroplasty showed a statistically significant reduction in rehospitalization rate in the intervention arm (3.4%; 95% CI, 0.1%-6.7%) compared with the usual care arm (12.2%; 95% CI, 6.4%-18.0%) ($P = .01$).[13] In a study of patients undergoing major abdominal surgery fitted with digital ankle pedometers yielding continuous measurements of their ambulation, there was a significant, independent inverse correlation between the number of steps on the first and second postoperative days (POD1/2) and the incidence of complications as well as the recovery of GI function and the likelihood of readmission ($P < .05$). POD2 step count was an independent risk factor for severe complications ($P = .026$).[14] These studies show promising effects of activity monitoring on surgical outcomes, which stands in contrast to a meta-analysis of RPM use in chronic medical conditions where difference-in-difference point estimation revealed no statistically significant impact on any of six reported clinical outcomes, including body mass index, weight, waist circumference, body fat percentage, systolic blood pressure, and diastolic blood pressure.[15] It is possible that the goal of preparing for, and recovering from a surgical intervention offers a discrete opportunity for patient-centered mHealth interventions with RPM, distinct from the long-term management of chronic medical diseases. Additionally, surgical outcomes of interest include post-procedure complications and health care utilization, not just physiologic measures, and offer a different paradigm to examine the impact of RPM. For example, use of a mobile app after major elective colorectal surgery was associated with fewer preventable emergency department visits (IRR 0.34, $P = .043$) and shorter length of stay (-1.62 days, $P = .011$).[16] In a randomized controlled trial of routine postoperative care compared with additional access to a smartphone-delivered wound assessment tool in patients undergoing emergency abdominal surgery, there was no significant difference in time-to-diagnosis of SSI for patients in the smartphone group, but they had 3.7-times higher odds of diagnosis within 7 postoperative days (95% CI: 1.02–13.51, P = .043). The smartphone group had significantly reduced community care attendance (OR: 0.57, 95% CI: 0.34–0.94, P = .030) and significantly better experiences in accessing care (OR: 2.02, 95% CI: 1.17–3.53, P = .013).[8] However, there are many other reports of less impactful RPM interventions, limited largely the implementation challenges. In a scoping review of abdominal surgery, continuous vital sign measurement and physical activity tracking both showed promise for detecting postoperative complications earlier than usual care, but conclusions were limited by poor device precision, adherence, occurrence of false alarms, data transmission problems, and retrospective data analysis.[17] Technology and methodological standards, as well as evaluative methods, are ever evolving, making it difficult to establish efficacy of surgical RPM.

Consideration for the specific needs of all stakeholders in the implementation and application of RPM is paramount. Sustained and effective use of symptom monitoring is dependent upon meeting the requirements of patients, care providers and administrators of health information systems, which may be in conflict.[18] Adopting RPM imposes a change to work process for the clinician, as patient-generated data submission requires review, acknowledgment and documentation. The patient experiences a change in their care process, as their data collection is required to drive the monitoring. This may require purchase, rental or loan of a new device such as a pulse oximeter, heart rate monitor or blood pressure cuff for recording and direct data transmission, or interaction with devices necessitating manual input of data at specified or demand intervals with response to electronic alerts. In addition, the patient is required to wear the device, comply with use guidelines (eg, keep it dry) and consent to data sharing. EHR-integrated systems are generally preferred by health care providers and organizations for security and usability concerns, but these are often associated with decreased patient usability and accessibility compared with standalone or proprietary systems marketed directly to patients. Patients generally want access to rapid expert assessment of their data and closed-loop communication, whereas providers want to limit data review to actionable (abnormal or concerning) data to make efficient and informed medical decisions, and HIT administrators want to limit security risk by maintaining closed and efficient EHR systems without customized add-ons. Compliance with RPM demands both patients and clinicians participate in the new monitoring process, as well as technology support for education and troubleshooting. Like other telehealth interventions, successful adoption and sustainability depends on an institutional commitment and the long-term impact of remote patient monitoring on the process of surgical care is unknown.

PATIENT- VERSUS PROVIDER-DRIVEN DIGITAL HEALTH

In contemplating the scope of digital health devices, apps and platforms, it is important to consider the intended focus. Some are patient-driven apps, created for preparation, self-tracking and self-improvement, whereas others are patient-focused, but driven by goals set from the provider perspective. Increasingly, the lines between digital health care and personal wellness are blurring, and the use of personal tracking in exercise, nutrition and education may be leveraged in the surgeon-patient relationship. Alternatively, self-tracking devices and apps may complicate the evaluation of a patient, as data sharing and interpretation can be frustrating. In this section, the patient-as-consumer-driven data acquisition is compared with that prescribed by providers in the context of surgical encounters.

Education for Patients Undergoing Surgery

Consumer-driven information seeking is increasingly apparent in initial surgical consultations. Patients now often arrive at initial visits for surgical consultation having performed Internet searches on provider bios and ratings, procedural options and disease prognosis. Access to previously restricted medical publications and videos of surgical procedures has exponentially increased with widespread use of the Internet for information sharing.

Surgery-specific patient educational materials with accessible language are available from trusted sources such as major medical centers and surgical organizations, but patients are left to curate their searches with little guidance, and the quality of information varies widely. For example, surgical procedures posted on YouTube are not vetted for safety or quality, and some are not content restricted.[19] Surgeons must address misinformation, misconceptions and unrealistic expectations as part of a digital health informed consent process.

In contrast, surgeon-driven educational tools leveraging mobile devices can more specifically direct pre- and postoperative patient education. A recent systematic review including both medical and surgical patients showed educating patients with timely medical information through their smartphones or tablets improves their levels of knowledge, medication or treatment adherence, satisfaction, and clinical outcomes, as well as having a positive effect on health care economics.[20] The effects were particularly seen when education was focused within a month of the medical or surgical encounter with a high frequency of engagement. A surgery-specific scoping review of apps designed to educate and evoke behavior change in the preoperative period was less conclusive, suggesting that some apps were more effective than others in preparing patients for surgery, and that standardization of outcome measures to evaluate adherence and educational effectiveness was important for future studies.[21] One digital health intervention, a perioperative, personalized Internet-based program which managed recovery expectations and provided postoperative guidance tailored to the patient after abdominal surgery, showed faster return to normal activities compared with usual care.

Median time until return to normal activities was 21 days (95% CI 17–25) in the intervention group and 26 days (20–32) in the control group (hazard ratio $1 \cdot 38$, 95% CI $1 \cdot 09$–$1 \cdot 73$; $P = 0 \cdot 007$). Complications did not differ between groups.[22,23] Although patient participants were overall satisfied with the intervention, the implementation scores of the different functions of the intervention were fair, with only 39% of approached subjects agreeing to participate. It is unclear how this digital health intervention would be accepted by patients in a real-world implementation outside of a research study.

Consumer Wellness versus Prescribed Prehabilitation and Early Recovery after Surgery

The consumer market for wellness apps and online platforms with device integration has exploded. The number of mHealth apps available to Android users via the Google Play Store reached over 65,300 thousand during the last quarter of 2021 and there were 52,406 health care and medical apps available on the Apple App Store, up by two percent compared with the previous quarter.[24,25] With increasing consumer demand for smartphones and smartwatches, and ease of use of Bluetooth-connected wearable devices such as heart rate monitors and activity trackers, self-tracking for fitness has reached a new level of acceptance. There has been a massive proliferation of consumer-directed wellness platforms, ranging from those targeting exercise activity tracking, to disseminating personalized weight loss recommendations, to promoting behavioral modifications for improving mental health. Although consumer use of mHealth apps and participation in wellness subscription platforms continues to grow, and there is evidence that use is associated with a higher level of physical activity,[26] their efficacy in sustained weight loss and improved cardiovascular fitness and mental health has not been established.[27] A major factor in the success of sustained platform use is the social networking engagement facilitated through associated web-based online communities.[28] Combining gamification elements of personalized goal setting and competition with active participation in the platform social network promotes sustained use and may effect better health outcomes, such as weight loss.[29] Increasingly, patients who use activity tracking wish to share their data in health care encounters, but this has not been adopted as a part of the standard preoperative risk assessment, which still relies on subjective report of patient mobility.

In contrast to those wellness apps and platforms directly targeting the patient as consumer, there have been a host of pilot studies of provider-prescribed digital health interventions intended to address optimization of health before and recovery after surgery. Interventions fall into the categories of prehabilitation, working to change behaviors to decrease modifiable preoperative risks, and early recovery after surgery (ERAS), targeting standard postoperative treatment pathways to improve time to discharge and return to baseline function. Automated text messaging interventions have been shown to be more effective than minimal smoking cessation support, but application of these interventions as part of surgical prehab is still in early phase testing.[30,31] A pilot study of a novel mobile device application for education and self-reporting of adherence for patients undergoing bowel surgery within an established early recovery program showed high agreement with traditional clinical audit, high usability, high patient satisfaction,[32] but a follow-up randomized trial of the same app did not result in improved adherence when compared with standard written patient education.[33] Even as these digital health tools take into account the educational needs of surgical patients, they are primarily designed from the surgeon's perspective, imposing standards agreed upon by expert consensus that were developed without patient input. A community-based prehabilitation model, with emphasis on shared-decision making and personal treatment recommendations, may offer a more comprehensive, patient-centered approach to care coordination along the whole surgical encounter.[34] Prescription of digital health services to support patients in preparation for and recovery from surgery is likely to be more acceptable to those who already employ self-tracking for wellness. As digital tracking becomes ever more present, while increasingly silent to consumers, there is potential to substantially change the patient experience with event-based alerts and guidance that facilitates personalized treatment.

CONSIDERATIONS AND CONTROVERSY

Adoption of digital health in surgical care has been relatively slower than in other areas of medicine. For example, in a systematic review to identify studies about RPM published between 2000 and 2018, cardiovascular disease was the topic of 47.8% of studies, whereas surgical pathologies and postoperative care represented only 2.6%.[35] Design and implementation of surgical digital health is linked to complex processes that require specific expertise in a wide array of data sources, data analytics, and clinical care delivery spanning the whole patient encounter, termed "surgical data science."[36] Patient empowerment has been slowed, mainly because of operational changes required to manage novel-patient-centered value-based interventions. Despite the appetite for innovation in surgery, there is a resistance to change patterns of care delivery.

Although patient satisfaction and convenience are improved with the adoption of telehealth, there is skepticism that digital health transformation will result in improved surgical outcomes. There is mistrust of "black box" methodology. Predictive analytics and recommendations derived from artificial intelligence algorithms are distinct from the traditional risk-based assessments performed by surgeons whose clinical decision-making is honed by accumulated personal experience. Additionally, the challenges of lack of interoperability of health information systems and integration of patient-generated health data have slowed the evolution of care, even as reimbursement of telehealth improved during the COVID-19 public health emergency.

Despite the ongoing consumer demand for telehealth services, there is real concern that reversion to more restrictive regulations of telehealth practice will further slow digital health transformation.

The return on the investment in adopting telehealth visits compared with in-person ambulatory care is clear for patients, with an avoidance of transportation costs, need for childcare, and lost wages/time from employment. Additionally, there is a positive environmental impact with avoidance of travel. Cost-effectiveness for the surgeon is perhaps more controversial, due to the lack of payment parity for telehealth encounters, but postoperative visits are already included within the bundled payment of the global period. There is an opportunity for more efficient clinic scheduling when telehealth is prioritized for postoperative follow-up care, with an increased new visit ratio, and availability for urgent in-person visits. A balance between serving the specific needs of patients and safe, efficient delivery of care is paramount. Further, a commitment to telehealth adoption and sustainability requires an investment in infrastructure and staffing, including technical support and education for both surgical providers and patients. The integration of digital health in a surgical practice goes beyond providing telehealth visits. Establishing an online reputation featuring a surgeon's scope of practice and curated patient education materials elevates the surgeon's profile in the competitive marketplace.

Usability and implementation challenges abound in the adoption of digital health services. Whether a surgical practice adopts an "off the shelf" digital health solution, or develops a customized intervention, successful implementation relies upon a commitment to the principles of user-centered design. The work process of both patients and surgical provider users must be taken into account. Bidirectional data transfer and communications are complicated because the needs, skills, and preferences of both sides of the conversation in the surgeon-patient relationship are different. In addition, adoption of a digital health solution does not ensure sustainability.

There are benefits to integration into an institutional EHR, including embedded privacy and security behind an established HIPAA-compliant firewall, but the tradeoff is time to develop and implement such systems, and the sacrifices that must be made to integrate into existing database structure and system visualizations. Use of lightweight and adaptable standalone apps as well as wellness platforms and devices already integrated into the patient's daily routine brings complexity to data transmission and documentation, but may increase the potential for durable use by patients. Patient adoption and sustained use may also be contingent upon their ownership of their own data, and their ability to opt in or out of data sharing, particularly after the surgical encounter has concluded.

As technology-based care continues to advance, equitable access to care is a major concern. The use of smartphones across populations served is dependent not only upon a patient's device access/ownership, but also their ability to use devices for purposes specific to surgical telemedicine, including RPM. Language, vision and other accessibility barriers pose additional challenges to providing telemedicine to all patients. Leveraging the patient's existing support network by involving their home care providers (eg, parents, adult children, in-home aides) in telehealth encounters may increase accessibility for pediatric and elderly patients, or others with communication or cognitive deficits. Some telehealth platforms provide translation services, or a translator may be conferenced in as a third party during a video visit. Connectivity may also be a problem for underserved populations. Many telehealth programs require a minimum of 1.5 Mbps for both upload and download speeds to successfully display audio and video data, and there are still locations in the United States, predominantly in rural areas, without stable broadband Internet access. Innovative devices such as hubs that allow Bluetooth wireless connected devices to transmit RPM data directly to the EHR via cellular network allow patients to avoid dependence on Wi-Fi or broadband. Systems for lending devices with return shipping to the care facility can enable successful short-term use of RPM, particularly for patients who live a considerable distance from the site providing services. Regional telehealth clinics where virtual consultations are facilitated may also serve as a bridge for patients without access to or facility with technology.

Finally, equitable care delivery requires more than just access to digital devices and programs. Diagnosis and treatment algorithms derived from majority populations have the potential to bias against minority populations, adversely impacting outcomes and exacerbating the gap in quality of care. An algorithm developed in one care facility without methods to account for generalizability may not perform with the same degree of accuracy in another facility with different patient characteristics. The use of heterogenous data sources to develop and refine algorithmic recommendations suitable for the characteristics of the patients served is essential to address disparities in care.

FUTURE DIRECTIONS

Effective dissemination of digital health to improve the surgical patient experience would be greatly facilitated by further development of standards, including quality assessment of existing apps, devices, and platforms. But a real digital transformation of care involves adopting a truly patient-centered approach to care delivery, adapting digital solutions already used widely in businesses such as banking and transportation that enable self-service.

Areas for future development include better integration of patient self-tracking practices and patient-generated data transmission to the EHR for shared decision-making and personalized treatment plans, as well as refining standards for automated versus provider-initiated communications. Dialogue systems (eg, chatbots) are widely used in business for triaging consumer-initiated online queries, and could serve to assist in patients finding their surgeon online, provide preoperative education about their surgical disease and operative options, as well as perform postoperative care triage.[37,38] Consumer fitness tracking platforms have shown that it is possible to take data uploads from multiple device sources and produce sophisticated visualizations of changes in physiology over time. Prehabilitation programs can produce similar data tracking for targeting weight loss, improved mobility, behavioral changes, and vital signs for optimization before surgery. Postoperative RPM is feasible with dashboard-based visualization and automated alert triggers to prioritize communications with patients exhibiting high-risk features suggestive of complications. A paradigm shift toward use of centralized telehealth providers and care coordination services may offload the monitoring burden on surgical providers and enable more efficient care delivery. These developments must take into account not only improving efficiency and quality, but also equity in access and treatment provision.

SUMMARY

The surgical patient experience is increasingly shaped by the adoption of digital health services. From patient-centered wellness programs leveraging self-tracking to institutionally based telemedicine platforms, the incorporation of apps, wearable devices, and new communication streams into surgical care is changing the way surgeons connect with their patients. Using patient-generated health data monitoring incorporated with patient-centered education and feedback, the promise of digital health is to optimally prepare patients for surgery and personalize postoperative care to improve not only clinical outcomes, but also quality of life. With continuous developments in technology and variable adoption, measuring the impact of digital health interventions on surgical outcomes brings new challenges and the need for adoption of new methods for implementation and evaluation. Equitable application of surgical digital health interventions includes considerations for accessibility as well as the development of new diagnostics and decision support that include the needs and characteristics of all populations served.

Dr H.L. Evans is a co-investigator: HRSA-FORHP Telehealth Center of Excellence Award (U66 RH31458).

CLINICS CARE POINTS

- A wide variety of wellness and health monitoring devices, apps, and platforms are marketed directly to the patient consumer. The quality of these programs varies widely, and the use by patients is variable.

- There is growing evidence that digital health services such as remote patient monitoring improve the patient experience, particularly in the postoperative phase. Surgeons should consider how preoperative education and postoperative care coordination may be impacted by the use of mHealth apps, patient portals, and integration of telehealth visits.

- Successful implementation of digital health interventions is dependent upon stakeholder engagement, collaboration, and user feedback integration. The needs of patients, surgeons, and health system administrators do not align uniformly, and these conflicts must be managed in order for digital health services to be sustainable beyond pilot programs.

REFERENCES

1. mHealth Economics 2017 Report: Status and trends in digital health | R2G [Internet]. research2guidance, 2017. Available at: https://research2guidance. com/product/mhealth-economics-2017-current-status-and-future-trends-in-mobile-health/ Accessed August 15, 2022.

2. Silver L, Huang C. 1. Social activities, information seeking on subjects like health and education top the list of mobile activities [Internet]. Pew Res Cent Internet Sci Tech 2019. Available at: https://www.pewresearch.org/internet/2019/08/22/social-activities-information-seeking-on-subjects-like-health-and-education-top-the-list-of-mobile-activities/. Accessed August 15, 2022.

3. Individuals' Access and Use of Patient Portals and Smartphone Health Apps, 2020 | HealthIT.gov [Internet]. Available at: https://www.healthit.gov/data/data-briefs/individuals-access-and-use-patient-portals-and-smartphone-health-apps-2020. Accessed August 15, 2022.

4. Harkey K, Connor CD, Wang H, et al. View from the patient perspective: mixed-methods analysis of post-discharge virtual visits in a randomized controlled trial. J Am Coll Surg 2021;233(5):593–605.e4.

5. Harkey K, Kaiser N, Zhao J, et al. Postdischarge virtual visits for low-risk surgeries: a randomized noninferiority clinical trial. JAMA Surg 2021;156(3):221–8.
6. Bray JO, Sutton TL, Akhter MS, et al. Telemedicine-based new patient consultations for hernia repair and advanced abdominal wall reconstruction. Hernia [Internet]. 2022. Available at: https://doi.org/10.1007/s10029-022-02624-8. Accessed August 15, 2022.
7. Telehealth for preoperative evaluation of patients with breast cancer during the COVID-19 pandemic | the permanente journal [Internet]. Available at: https://www.thepermanentejournal.org/doi/full/10.7812/TPP/21.126. Accessed August 15, 2022.
8. McLean KA, Mountain KE, Shaw CA, et al, TWIST Collaborators. Remote diagnosis of surgical-site infection using a mobile digital intervention: a randomised controlled trial in emergency surgery patients. NPJ Digit Med 2021;4(1):160.
9. Wang T, Stanforth PR, Fleming RYD, et al. A mobile app with multimodality prehabilitation programs for patients awaiting elective surgery: development and usability study. JMIR Perioper Med 2021;4(2):e32575.
10. Atilgan K, Onuk BE, Köksal Coşkun P, et al. Remote patient monitoring after cardiac surgery: the utility of a novel telemedicine system. J Cardiovasc Surg 2021; 36(11):4226–34.
11. Fleming JN, Pollock MD, Taber DJ, et al. Review and evaluation of mhealth apps in solid organ transplantation: past, present, and future. Transpl Direct 2022;8(3): e1298.
12. Dawes AJ, Lin AY, Varghese C, et al. Mobile health technology for remote home monitoring after surgery: a meta-analysis. Br J Surg 2021;108(11):1304–14.
13. Mehta SJ, Hume E, Troxel AB, et al. Effect of remote monitoring on discharge to home, return to activity, and rehospitalization after hip and knee arthroplasty: a randomized clinical trial. JAMA Netw Open 2020;3(12):e2028328.
14. Nevo Y, Shaltiel T, Constantini N, et al. Activity tracking after surgery: does it correlate with postoperative complications? Am Surg 2022;88(2):226–32.
15. Noah B, Keller MS, Mosadeghi S, et al. Impact of remote patient monitoring on clinical outcomes: an updated meta-analysis of randomized controlled trials. Npj Digit Med 2018;1(1):1–12.
16. Eustache J, Latimer EA, Liberman S, et al. A mobile phone app improves patient-physician communication and reduces emergency department visits after colorectal surgery. Dis Colon Rectum 2021. https://doi.org/10.1097/DCR.0000000000002187.
17. Wells CI, Xu W, Penfold JA, et al. Wearable devices monitor recovery after abdominal surgery: scoping review. BJS Open 2022;6(2):zrac031.
18. Sanger PC, Hartzler A, Lordon RJ, et al. A patient-centered system in a provider-centered world: challenges of incorporating post-discharge wound data into practice. J Am Med Inform Assoc JAMIA 2016;23(3):514–25.
19. Jackson HT, Hung CMS, Potarazu D, et al. Attending guidance advised: educational quality of surgical videos on YouTube. Surg Endosc 2022;36(6):4189–98.
20. Timmers T, Janssen L, Kool RB, et al. Educating patients by providing timely information using smartphone and tablet apps: systematic review. J Med Internet Res 2020;22(4):e17342.
21. Åsberg K, Bendtsen M. Perioperative digital behaviour change interventions for reducing alcohol consumption, improving dietary intake, increasing physical activity and smoking cessation: a scoping review. Perioper Med (Lond) 2021;10(1):18.
22. van der Meij E, Anema JR, Leclercq WKG, et al. Personalized perioperative care by e-health after intermediate-grade abdominal surgery: a multicenter, single-blind, randomised, placebo-controlled trial. Lancet 2018;392(10141):51–9.

23. Meij van der E, Huirne JA, Bouwsma EV, et al. Substitution of usual perioperative care by ehealth to enhance postoperative recovery in patients undergoing general surgical or gynecological procedures: study protocol of a randomized controlled trial. JMIR Res Protoc 2016;5(4):e6580.

24. Healthcare apps available Apple App Store 2022 [Internet]. Statista. Available at: https://www.statista.com/statistics/779910/health-apps-available-ios-worldwide/. Accessed August 21, 2022.

25. Healthcare apps available Google Play 2022 [Internet]. Statista. Available at: https://www.statista.com/statistics/779919/health-apps-available-google-play-worldwide/. Accessed August 21, 2022.

26. Petersen JM, Kemps E, Lewis LK, et al. Cross-sectional study. J Med Internet Res 2020;22(6):e17152.

27. Romeo A, Edney S, Plotnikoff R, et al. Can smartphone apps increase physical activity? systematic review and meta-analysis. J Med Internet Res 2019;21(3):e12053.

28. Petersen JM, Prichard I, Kemps E. A comparison of physical activity mobile apps with and without existing web-based social networking platforms: systematic review. J Med Internet Res 2019;21(8):e12687.

29. Yang H, Li D. Health management gamification: understanding the effects of goal difficulty, achievement incentives, and social networks on performance. Technol Forecast Soc Change 2021;169:120839.

30. Thomas K, Bendtsen M, Linderoth C, et al. Implementing facilitated access to a text messaging, smoking cessation intervention among swedish patients having elective surgery: qualitative study of patients' and health care professionals' perspectives. JMIR MHealth UHealth 2020;8(9):e17563.

31. Bendtsen M, Linderoth C, Bendtsen P. Mobile phone–based smoking-cessation intervention for patients undergoing elective surgery: protocol for a randomized controlled trial. JMIR Res Protoc 2019;8(3):e12511.

32. Pecorelli N, Fiore JF, Kaneva P, et al. An app for patient education and self-audit within an enhanced recovery program for bowel surgery: a pilot study assessing validity and usability. Surg Endosc 2018;32(5):2263–73.

33. Mata J, Pecorelli N, Kaneva P, et al. A mobile device application (app) to improve adherence to an enhanced recovery program for colorectal surgery: a randomized controlled trial. Surg Endosc 2020;34(2):742–51.

34. Barberan-Garcia A, Cano I, Bongers BC, et al. Digital support to multimodal community-based prehabilitation: looking for optimization of health value generation. Front Oncol 2021;11. Available at: https://www.frontiersin.org/articles/10.3389/fonc.2021.662013. Accessed July 9, 2022.

35. Farias FAC, Dagostini CM, Bicca YA, et al. Remote patient monitoring: a systematic review. Telemed J E Health 2020;26(5):576–83.

36. Vedula SS, Hager GD. Surgical data science: the new knowledge domain. Innov Surg Sci 2017;2(3):109–21.

37. Lordon RJ. Design, development, and evaluation of a patient-centered health dialog system to support inguinal hernia surgery patient information-seeking [Internet] [Thesis]. 2019. Available at: https://digital.lib.washington.edu:443/researchworks/handle/1773/44675. Accessed August 21, 2022.

38. Geoghegan L, Scarborough A, Wormald JCR, et al. Automated conversational agents for post-intervention follow-up: a systematic review. BJS Open 2021;5(4):zrab070.

Moving?

Make sure your subscription moves with you!

To notify us of your new address, find your **Clinics Account Number** (located on your mailing label above your name), and contact customer service at:

Email: journalscustomerservice-usa@elsevier.com

800-654-2452 (subscribers in the U.S. & Canada)
314-447-8871 (subscribers outside of the U.S. & Canada)

Fax number: 314-447-8029

**Elsevier Health Sciences Division
Subscription Customer Service
3251 Riverport Lane
Maryland Heights, MO 63043**

*To ensure uninterrupted delivery of your subscription, please notify us at least 4 weeks in advance of move.

Printed and bound by CPI Group (UK) Ltd, Croydon, CR0 4YY

16/10/2024

01774832-0001